$19.95

STROKE ESSENTIALS

Adrian J. Goldszmidt, MD
Director, Cerebrovascular Program
Sinai Hospital
Instructor of Neurology
Johns Hopkins School of Medicine
Baltimore, Maryland

Louis R. Caplan, MD
Director of Cerebrovascular Disease
Beth Israel Deaconess Medical Cente
Professor of Neurology
Harvard Medical School
Boston, Massachusetts

PHYSICIANS' PRESS

www.physicianspress.com

616.8
GOL
2003

ABOUT THE AUTHORS

Adrian J. Goldszmidt, MD, is Director of the Cerebrovascular Disorders Program at Sinai Hospital and Instructor in Neurology at Johns Hopkins University Medical School, Baltimore, Maryland. After completing medical school at Harvard, he trained in Neurology at Harvard's Longwood program in Boston, then did a stroke fellowship at New England Medical Center. Dr. Goldszmidt has been an investigator in numerous acute stroke trials and has research interests in platelet function in stroke. He is actively involved in patient care.

Louis R. Caplan, MD, is Director of Cerebrovascular Disease, Beth Israel Deaconess Medical Center, Boston, Massachusetts; Professor of Neurology, Harvard Medical School, Boston, Massachusetts; and one of the world's leading authorities on stroke. During his distinguished career, he served as Chair of the Neurology Department at Beth Israel Hospital in Boston, Neurologist-in-Chief at Michael Reese Hospital in Chicago and the New England Medical Center in Boston, Professor of Neurology at the University of Chicago, and Professor and Chairman of the Department of Neurology and Professor of Medicine at Tufts Medical Center in Boston. He also served as Chairman of the Stroke Council of the American Heart Association and as chair of numerous neurological and stroke organizations. At Beth Israel Hospital, he founded the Harvard Stroke Registry. He is a diplomat of both the American Board of Internal Medicine and the American Board of Neurology and Psychiatry. He is the author or editor of 26 books, including the landmark textbook, *Stroke: A Clinical Approach*, now in its 3rd edition, and he has contributed more than 500 scholarly articles to the medical literature. He also serves or has served on the editorial board of 21 medical journals. He speaks nationally and internationally on stroke and has delivered 18 named lectureships, including the 2000 Thomas Willis lecture for the American Heart Association. Dr.Caplan has received several teaching awards as well as the Distinguished Achievement Award from the American Heart Association.

Copyright © 2003
Physicians' Press

Additional copies of *Stroke Essentials* can be obtained at medical bookstores or by contacting:

Physicians' Press
620 Cherry Avenue
Royal Oak, Michigan, 48073
(248) 616-3023 / fax: (248) 616-3003
www.physicianspress.com

Printed in the United States of America   ISBN: 1-890114-45-6

*For stroke patients now
and in the future*

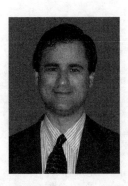

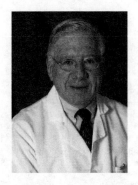

Adrian J. Goldszmidt, MD   Louis R. Caplan, MD

TABLE OF CONTENTS

ACKNOWLEDGMENTS

To accomplish the task of presenting the data compiled in this reference, a small, dedicated team of professionals was assembled. This team focused their energy and discipline for many months into typing, revising, designing, illustrating, and formatting the many chapters that comprise this text. We wish to acknowledge Rebecca Smith and Monica Crowder-Kaufmann for their important contribution. We would also like to thank Drs. Kaplan, Weber, Ballantyne, O'Keefe, and Gotto for graciously contributing their time and energy amidst busy professional lives, Norman Lyle for cover design, and Mark S. Freed, MD, President and Editor-in-Chief of Physicians' Press, for his vision, commitment, and guidance.

Adrian J. Goldszmidt, MD
Louis R. Caplan, MD

NOTICE

CONTRIBUTORS

Christie M. Ballantyne, MD
Clinical Director, Section of
Atherosclerosis
Professor of Medicine
Baylor College of Medicine
Director, Center for Cardiovascular
Disease Prevention
Methodist DeBakey Heart Center
Houston, Texas
Dyslipidemia and Risk Reduction

Louis R. Caplan, MD
Director of Cerebrovascular Disease
Beth Israel Deaconess Medical Center
Professor of Neurology
Harvard Medical School
Boston, Massachusetts

Adrian J. Goldszmidt, MD
Director, Cerebrovascular Program
Sinai Hospital
Instructor of Neurology
Johns Hopkins School of Medicine
Baltimore, Maryland

Mark S. Freed, MD
Cardiologist
President and Editor-in-Chief
Physicians' Press
Royal Oak, Michigan
Hypertension and Risk Reduction

Antonio M. Gotto, Jr, MD, DPhil
The Stephen and Suzanne Weiss Dean
Professor of Medicine
Provost for Medical Affairs
The Weill Medical College of Cornell University
New York, New York
Dyslipidemia and Risk Reduction

Norman M. Kaplan, MD
Professor of Medicine
University of Texas Southwestern Medical
Center
Dallas, Texas
Hypertension and Risk Reduction

James H. O'Keefe, Jr, MD
Director, Preventive Cardiology
Mid America Heart Institute
Clinical Professor of Medicine
University of Missouri School of Medicine
Kansas City, Missouri
Dyslipidemia and Risk Reduction

Michael A. Weber, MD
Professor of Medicine
Associate Dean
SUNY Downstate College of Medicine
Brooklyn, New York
Hypertension and Risk Reduction

ABBREVIATIONS

ABC	airway, breathing, circulation	ICH	intracerebral hemorrhage
ACA	anterior cerebral artery	IV	intravenous
ACC	American College of Cardiology	kg	kilogram
ACE	angiotensin converting enzyme	L	liter
ACS	acute coronary syndrome	LDL	low-density lipoprotein
AHA	American Heart Association	LP	lumbar puncture
ATP	Adult Treatment Panel (National Cholesterol Education Program)	LV	left ventricular; left ventricle
		max	maximum
AV	arteriovenous	MCA	middle cerebral artery
BAS	bile acid sequestrants	mcg	microgram
BID	twice daily	mcL	microliter
BMI	body mass index	mg	milligram
BP	blood pressure	MI	myocardial infarction
BUN	blood urea nitrogen	min	minute
CABG	coronary artery bypass grafting	mL	milliliter
CEA	carotid endarterectomy	MRA	magnetic resonance angiography
CHD	coronary heart disease	MRI	magnetic resonance imaging
CI	contraindication	NCEP	National Cholesterol Education Program
CK	creatine kinase		
CNS	central nervous system	NHLBI	National Heart, Lung, and Blood Institute
COPD	chronic obstructive pulmonary disease		
CrCl	creatinine clearance	NPO	nothing by mouth
CT	computerized tomography	NRT	nicotine replacement therapy
CTA	CT angiography	O_2	oxygen
DHA	docosahexaenoic acid	PCA	posterior cerebral artery
dL	deciliter	PCOM	posterior communication artery
ECG	electrocardiogram	PE	pulmonary embolism
Echo	echocardiogram; echocardiography	PO	per os - by mouth; oral
EF	ejection fraction	PT	prothrombin time
e.g.	for example	PTT	partial thromboplastin time
EPA	eicosapentaenoic acid	q__h	every __ hours
FDA	Food and Drug Administration	q__d	every __ days
g	gram	SAH	subarachnoid hemorrhage
GI	gastrointestinal	TIA	transient ischemic attack
gm	gram	TID	three times daily
HDL	high-density lipoprotein	TLC	therapeutic lifestyle changes
ICA	internal carotid artery	tPA	tissue plasminogen activator

DIAGNOSIS, EVALUATION, AND TREATMENT OF STROKE

Chapter 1

Overview of Stroke

Stroke is the third most common cause of death in developed countries behind cardiovascular disease and cancer. Each year, more than 700,000 Americans develop strokes, 25% of whom are under age 65, and 150,000 people die from stroke or its immediate complications. At any one time, 4.7 million people in the United States have had strokes, resulting in stroke-related health care costs in excess of $18 billion per year. Stroke is broadly classified into ischemic and hemorrhagic stroke (Figure 1.1, Table 1.1). Ischemic stroke accounts for 80% of strokes and is subdivided into large artery atherothrombosis, brain embolism, lacunar stroke, and systemic hypoperfusion (Chapter 2). Brain hemorrhage accounts for the remaining 20% of strokes and is subdivided into intracerebral hemorrhage, subarachnoid hemorrhage, and subdural/extradural hematoma (Chapter 4). The distinction between ischemic stroke and hemorrhagic stroke is crucial: Early, appropriate use of thrombolytic therapy reduces the risk of moderate or severe disability by 30% in ischemic stroke but is contraindicated in hemorrhagic stroke, where it would exacerbate the problem. For every 100 patients treated with intravenous tissue plasminogen activator (tPA), at least 11 additional patients will have a favorable outcome over the following year (Chapter 3). Aggressive management of stroke-related complications (Chapter 5) and consistent application of cerebrovascular and cardiovascular risk reduction measures (Chapters 8-13) are also important for prognosis.

Stroke Essentials provides a concise, authoritative, and practical guide to the detection, evaluation, and treatment of stroke. Primary and secondary prevention measures are also emphasized, forming the basis for a management strategy aimed at halting the progression of atherosclerosis, stabilizing rupture-prone plaques, preventing arterial thromboembolism, and improving prognosis. The initial evaluation and management of stroke are summarized in Figure 1.2.

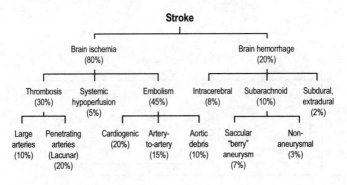

Figure 1.1. Classification of Stroke

Table 1.1. Ischemic vs. Hemorrhagic Stroke: General Features

	Ischemic Stroke	Hemorrhagic Stroke
Incidence	80% of strokes	20% of strokes
Patho-physiology	Large artery atherothrombosis; brain embolism; intracranial atherosclerosis; lipohyalinosis of small, penetrating vessels	Rupture of berry aneurysm, AV malformation; severe hypertension; bleeding diathesis; trauma
Presentation	Neurological deficit usually in distribution of one vascular territory. TIA in 30-50%. Headache, decreased consciousness uncommon	Neurological deficit not necessarily limited to one vascular territory. TIA uncommon. Headache, vomiting, decreased consciousness common
Initial treatment	Large artery atherothrombosis: tPA within 3 hours; otherwise aspirin Cardiogenic embolism: tPA within 3 hours; otherwise heparin Lacunar stroke: empiric antiplatelet therapy, control of blood pressure	Subarachnoid hemorrhage: clipping, coiling, coating, or trapping of berry aneurysm (early); excision or embolization of AV malformation (late); nimodipine to prevent vasospasm Intracerebral hemorrhage: control of hypertension, bleeding diatheses; surgical drainage of large hematomas Subdural/extradural hematoma: surgical drainage if large

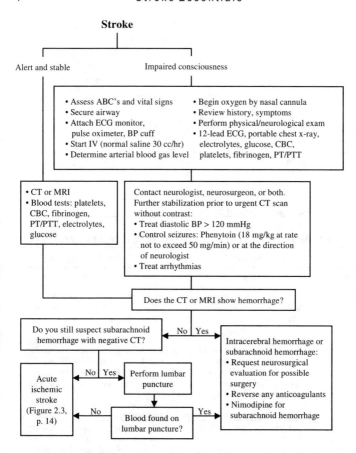

Figure 1.2. Initial Evaluation and Management of Stroke

ABC = airway, breathing, circulation, BP = blood pressure, CBC = complete blood count, CT = computerized tomography, ECG = electrocardiogram, MRI = magnetic resonance imaging, PT/PTT = prothrombin time/partial thromboplastin time

Detection and Evaluation of Stroke

A. **History, Physical Examination, Laboratory Testing.** Acute ischemic stroke presents with sudden onset of a focal neurological deficit of presumed vascular origin. The diagnosis requires exclusion of brain hemorrhage and nonvascular mimics: seizure with postictal neurologic deficit, subdural hematoma, brain tumor, brain abscess, encephalitis, complicated migraine, glucose abnormalities. The primary purpose of the initial evaluation is to identify the type of stroke (ischemic or hemorrhagic) and to determine whether the patient is eligible for thrombolytic or other therapy. Lytic therapy is usually reserved for patients with onset of ischemic stroke within 3 hours in the absence of cerebral hemorrhage or other exclusion criteria (Table 3.1, p. 28). Although not approved for this indication, thrombolytic therapy is sometimes administered 3-6 hours after stroke onset if diffusion/perfusion-weighted MRI and MRA show arterial occlusion with no or minor brain infarction and a large brain area that is underperfused but not yet infarcted. When the occlusion involves the basilar artery, intra-arterial thrombolysis may be successful even after 12-18 hours of ischemia. The initial history and physical examination are also used to assess the extent of neurological dysfunction and to identify risk factors for atherothrombosis and comorbid medical conditions (Table 1.2). Laboratory testing is used to identify a potential cause of stroke (e.g., hyperviscosity syndrome, coagulopathy), to detect stroke-related complications (e.g., hyponatremia due to SiADH), to establish baseline coagulation parameters, and to identify risk factors for generalized atherosclerosis (e.g., dyslipidemia). Vascular imaging (MRA, CTA, ultrasound) is used to detect the presence and location of occlusive thromboemboli.

Table 1.2. Clinical Evaluation of the Stroke Patient

History
- Past history of stroke or TIA; time of onset of symptoms; activity at time of stroke; temporal progression of symptoms (e.g., maximal at onset, gradual worsening, worsening in step-like fashion)
- Accompanying signs: headache, neck pain, vomiting, decreased consciousness
- Risk factors/history of vascular disease: hypertension, dyslipidemia, myocardial infarction, angina, palpitations, rheumatic heart disease, heart failure, aortic aneurysm, peripheral arterial disease, smoking, diabetes mellitus
- Nonatherosclerotic conditions associated with focal neurological deficit: history of seizures, migraine, brain tumor, cerebral aneurysm, head trauma, multiple sclerosis, blood dyscrasia, illicit drug use

Physical Examination
- Vital signs; neurological exam
- HEENT exam for head trauma, retinal changes (hypertensive, cholesterol crystals, papilledema, subhyaloid hemorrhage)
- Neck exam for bruits
- Heart exam for murmurs, gallops, ventricular dysfunction, pulmonary hypertension
- Abdominal exam for bruits, aneurysm
- Peripheral vascular exam for bruits, decreased pulses, ischemic skin changes

Laboratory Testing
- Complete blood count to identify potential cause of stroke: hematocrit > 60%; WBC > 150,000/mm^3; platelets > 1 million/mm^3 or < 20,000/mm^3; evidence of sickle cell anemia or other hemoglobinopathies
- Sedimentation rate (elevated in tumor, infection, vasculitis)
- Serum glucose (hyperglycemia may worsen acute outcome; hypoglycemia may cause focal neurological changes)
- Electrolytes
- Lipid profile and fibrinogen
- PT, PTT, and INR to detect coagulopathies and for use as a baseline prior to anticoagulation therapy
- Anticardiolipin antibodies
- RPR for neurosyphilis
- Urine screen for cocaine, if suspected

B. Imaging. All patients with suspected stroke should have an emergency unenhanced CT scan or MRI to differentiate ischemic from hemorrhagic stroke and to identify tumor or mass effect (suggesting large stroke). Ischemic stroke is the most likely diagnosis when the CT scan does not show hemorrhage, tumor, or focal infection, and the clinical findings do not suggest migraine, hypoglycemia, encephalitis, or subarachnoid hemorrhage.

1. **CT/MRI**

   CT/MRI is used to determine the location, type (ischemia or hemorrhage), and complications of stroke (edema, mass effect, hydrocephalus). It is also used to exclude nonvascular causes of neurological symptoms (tumors, hydrocephalus). MRI is more sensitive than CT scan for detecting brain infarction within the first 72 hours and for evaluating the posterior fossa (brainstem and cerebellum), but CT can better differentiate hemorrhage from ischemia in acute lesions. Diffusion/perfusion-weighted MRI is particularly useful in identifying infarcted brain and underperfused brain regions at risk for infarction if reperfusion does not occur. Sensitivity of the CT scan for detecting subarachnoid blood drops from 90% on day 1 to 50% at one week. Lumbar puncture is required for suspected subarachnoid hemorrhage in patients with a normal CT.

2. **Doppler ultrasound.** Duplex ultrasound is warranted to assess stenosis or occlusion of the carotid and vertebral arteries in the neck. The transcranial approach can be used to assess the direction and velocity of blood flow in the circle of Willis and to identify vascular lesions in both anterior and posterior circulations.

3. **Magnetic Resonance Angiography.** MRA is used to screen for severe occlusive disease of extracranial arteries and intracranial large arteries. It is also used to screen for aneurysms in patients with a predisposition (e.g., fibromuscular dysplasia, polycystic kidneys). Computed tomography angiography (CTA) is less prone to artifact from turbulence or complex flow patterns than MRA.

4. **Cerebral angiography.** Angiography is used to define the nature, location and severity of vascular occlusive disease, and to identify vascular abnormalities leading to brain hemorrhage (saccular

aneurysm, AV malformation). Cerebral angiography is best used in conjunction with brain imaging (CT, MRI) and non-invasive vascular screening modalities (ultrasound, MRA, CTA).

5. **Lumbar puncture.** Lumbar puncture (LP) is used to diagnose subarachnoid hemorrhage when CT/MRI are unavailable or negative (i.e., when bleeding is minor or several days old); the absence of blood on LP excludes the diagnosis of subarachnoid hemorrhage. LP is also important when CNS infection (meningitis, meningovascular syphilis) is suspected.

6. **Echocardiogram.** Echocardiography is used to assess the nature and extent of myocardial/valvular disease when cardiogenic embolism is suspected as the etiology of stroke. Transesophageal echo is more sensitive than transthoracic echo for the detection of aortic atherothrombotic debris, aortic dissection, atrial septal aneurysms, left atrial clot, infectious endocarditis, and shunts.

7. **Electrocardiography.** The electrocardiogram is used to detect myocardial ischemia/infarction, arrhythmias, and chamber enlargement suggesting cardiomyopathy or valvular heart disease.

8. **Holter monitoring.** Ambulatory ECG monitoring is used to detect paroxysmal arrhythmia when suspected as a cause of cardiogenic embolism.

9. **Electroencephalography.** EEG is useful for suspected seizures but not for clarification of stroke subtype or stroke severity.

Chapter 2

Ischemic Stroke

Eighty percent of strokes are ischemic in origin and are caused by thrombotic or thromboembolic arterial occlusion. The most common sites of clot origin include the extracranial cerebral arteries, the heart (atrial fibrillation, mitral valve disease, left ventricular thrombus), the small penetrating arteries of the brain (lacunar stroke), and aortic arch plaque (Figure 2.1). Ischemic stroke is subdivided into large artery atherothrombosis, brain embolism, lacunar stroke, and systemic hypoperfusion (Table 2.1). Ischemic stroke typically presents as a focal neurological deficit in the distribution of a single blood vessel (Figure 2.2). Findings can wax and wane, and there may be a progressive worsening or stepwise deterioration in neurologic function. Vomiting and loss of consciousness are rare.

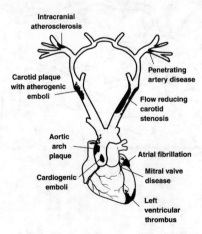

Figure 2.1. Common Sites and Mechanisms of Ischemic Stroke

Adapted from: Sixth ACCP Consensus Conference on Antithrombotic Therapy. Chest 2001;119:300S-230S

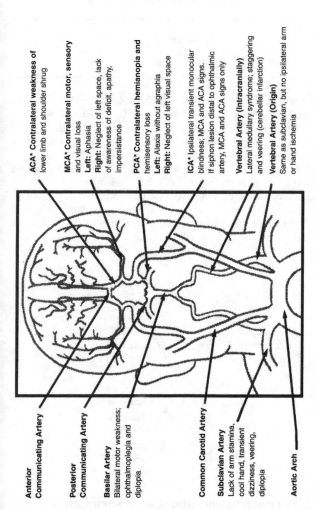

Anterior Communicating Artery

Posterior Communicating Artery

Basilar Artery
Bilateral motor weakness; ophthalmoplegia and diplopia

Common Carotid Artery

Subclavian Artery
Lack of arm stamina, cool hand, transient dizziness, veering, diplopia

Aortic Arch

ACA* Contralateral weakness of lower limb and shoulder shrug

MCA* Contralateral motor, sensory and visual loss
Left: Aphasia
Right: Neglect of left space, lack of awareness of deficit, apathy, impersistance

PCA* Contralateral hemianopia and hemisensory loss
Left: Alexia without agraphia
Right: Neglect of left visual space

ICA* Ipsilateral transient monocular blindness; MCA and ACA signs. If siphon lesion distal to ophthalmic artery, MCA and ACA signs only

Vertebral Artery (Intracranially)
Lateral medullary syndrome; staggering and veering (cerebellar infarction)

Vertebral Artery (Origin)
Same as subclavian, but no ipsilateral arm or hand ischemia

Figure 2.2. Clinical Presentation of Common Stroke Syndromes

ACA = anterior cerebral artery, ICA = internal carotid artery, MCA = middle cerebral artery, PCA = posterior cerebral artery

Table 2.1. Ischemic Stroke: Clinical Features

	Large Artery Thrombosis	Brain Embolism	Lacunar Infarct	Hypoperfusion
Risk factors	Smoking, coronary artery disease, dyslipidemia, diabetes, males, peripheral arterial disease	Atrial fibrillation, valvular disease, LV thrombus, cardiomyopathy, coronary artery disease, aortic arch plaque	Hypertension, diabetes, polycythemia	All forms of shock
Onset of neurologic deficit	Preceded by TIAs in 50%. Often occurs during sleep (i.e., patient awakes with neurological deficit). Neurologic changes often fluctuate in a stepwise progressive or remitting fashion, due to recanalization, re-thrombosis, and changes in collateral blood flow	Sudden in 80%, with maximal deficit at onset. Others show stepwise progression during the first 24 hours. Middle cerebral artery syndrome is the most common presentation: contralateral sensorimotor deficit (arm/face > leg), aphasia (dominant hemisphere), unawareness of deficit (non-dominant hemisphere) ± quadrantanopsia	Fluctuating, progressive stepwise, or remitting. May gradually worsen over hours to days. Preceded by TIAs in 25%. Several distinct lacunar syndromes (p. 24)	Begins with systemic disorder

Table 2.1. Ischemic Stroke: Clinical Features

	Large Artery Thrombosis	Brain Embolism	Lacunar Infarct	Hypoperfusion
Associated symptoms	Headache before, at, or after onset. Vomiting, loss of consciousness are rare	Neurologic deficit is usually maximal at onset. Headache at or after onset. Vomiting, decreased consciousness are uncommon	Usually none (i.e., alert without headache or vomiting)	Pallor, sweating, hypotension
Stroke location	Superficial cortex (most often middle cerebral artery), cerebellum, or territory of posterior cerebral artery	Same as for large artery thrombosis	Deep brain structures (basal ganglia, cerebral white matter, thalamus, pons, cerebellum)	Border zone between anterior, middle, and posterior cerebral arteries, or between posteroinferior, anteroinferior, and superior cerebellar arteries
Imaging	CT: low density lesion (dark). May take hours to days before scan becomes positive MRI: dark (T1-weighted images); bright (T2-weighted images). Able to demonstrate abnormality within hours of infarction	CT: low-density lesion (dark) MRI: dark (T1-weighted images); bright (T2-weighted images). Wedge shaped; superficial only or superficial and deep	CT: low-density (dark) MRI: dark (T1-weighted images); bright (T2-weighted images). Small, deep lesions	CT: low density lesion (dark) MRI: dark (T1-weighted images); bright (T2-weighted images)

Table 2.1. Ischemic Stroke: Clinical Features

	Large Artery Thrombosis	Brain Embolism	Lacunar Infarct	Hypoperfusion
Treatment	Thrombolytic therapy for onset < 3 hours. Aspirin ± heparin for others. Carotid endarterectomy (or stenting) for moderate or severe stenosis	Warfarin, aspirin, antiarrhythmic, aneurysmectomy, repair of atrial septal defect, or resection of atrial myxoma, depending on source of embolism	Long-term control of hypertension ± antiplatelet therapy. Maintenance of blood pressure acutely	Maintenance of blood pressure with fluids, vasopressors, intra-aortic balloon pump until specific therapy can be instituted
Prognosis	Mortality 20% at 1 month and 25% at 1 year. Two-thirds of survivors lead an independent existence. Thrombolytic therapy reduces significant disability by 30%. Early cause of death is herniation (< 72 hours) and cardiac disease or sepsis (> 72 hours). Recovery of language/motor function is unlikely if no improvement within 2 weeks. Neurologic deficits beyond 6 months usually persist	If embolism is cardiogenic in origin, 10-15% develop a second embolus within 2 weeks	Prognosis is good for recovery of function. Other lacunes frequently develop	Prognosis depends on severity of hypotension. Most who eventually recover awaken by 72 hours. Adverse prognostic factors include dilated non-reactive pupils >12 hours and absent corneal, oculocephalic, oculovestibular reflexes

Overview of Treatment of Ischemic Stroke

Initial treatment of ischemic stroke depends on the type of stroke and eligibility for thrombolytic therapy (Figure 2.3). Measures to prevent recurrent stroke are based on the location/severity of the stenosis (Table 2.2) or the presumed embolic source (Table 2.3).

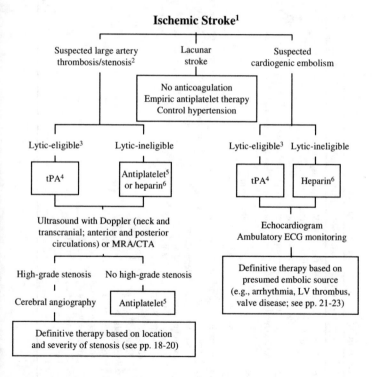

Figure 2.3. Evaluation and Treatment of Ischemic Stroke

See footnotes, next page

<u>Footnotes for Figure 2.3</u>
MRA/CTA = magnetic resonance angiogram/computed tomography angiogram

1. Absence of intracranial or subarachnoid hemorrhage on CT or MRI and exclusion of nonvascular mimics (seizure with postictal neurologic deficit, subdural hematoma, brain tumor, brain abscess, encephalitis, complicated migraine, glucose abnormalities).

2. Innominate, common carotid, internal carotid, vertebral, basilar, anterior cerebral, middle cerebral, or posterior cerebral arteries.

3. Less than 3 hours from symptom onset; no hemorrhage on CT scan; early infarct not more than 1/3 of middle cerebral artery territory; no exclusion criteria (Table 3.1). Although not approved for this indication, tPA may be considered 3-6 hours after stroke onset if the diffusion/perfusion MRI demonstrates vascular occlusion with no or minor infarction and a large brain area that is underperfused but not yet infarcted, under the guidance of a neurologist.

4. tPA 0.9 mg/kg total (maximum 90 mg): 10% of total dose as IV bolus over 1 minute followed by remaining 90% as a constant IV infusion over 60 minutes. Anticoagulants and antiplatelet agents are withheld x 24 hours.

5. Either aspirin 160-325 mg once daily, clopidogrel 75 mg once daily, or combination low-dose aspirin 25 mg plus extended-release dipyridamole 200 mg twice daily, in patients not receiving heparin, starting within 48 hours of stroke onset. See discussion, pp. 77-85.

6. Given the high risk of stroke progression or recurrence, it is reasonable to administer IV heparin acutely to lytic-ineligible patients if either: (1) vascular imaging or echocardiography identifies a cardiac source of embolism or a recent occlusion/severe stenosis of a large extracranial or intracranial artery; or (2) a cardiac source of embolism or large artery atherothrombosis is suspected clinically, until vascular imaging and echocardiography are performed. All other lytic-ineligible patients and those with a contraindication to heparin (a large brain infarct is a relative contraindication) should be treated with aspirin 160-325 mg/d or another antiplatelet agent, starting within 48 hours of stroke onset. Unfractionated heparin should be given as an IV infusion (without bolus) starting at 800-1000 U/hr and adjusted to maintain the PTT at 1.5-2.5 times control until a mechanism of stroke is identified and more definitive treatment is instituted. Low-molecular-weight heparin reduced mortality in one randomized trial (p. 118) but is not yet approved for use in stroke in the U.S.

Lytic-Eligible Patients

When used in strict accordance with the National Institute of Neurological Diseases and Stroke (NINDS) tPA study protocol, IV administration of tPA within 3 hours of stroke onset increases the likelihood of minimal or no disability by 30% or more. Inclusion and exclusion criteria, baseline evaluation, dosing and administration guidelines, management of complications, and post-lytic measures are described in Chapter 3.

Lytic-Ineligible Patients

Despite the efficacy of thrombolytic therapy for acute ischemic stroke caused by large artery atherothrombosis or brain embolism, more than 95% of patients fail to meet eligibility criteria for thrombolysis, usually due to late presentation. For this large group of patients, therapy consists of aspirin or heparin. In some investigational centers, mechanical removal of thrombus (e.g., AngioJet) and acute angioplasty with stenting are being applied.

A. Antiplatelet Therapy. All lytic-ineligible patients not treated with IV heparin should receive antiplatelet therapy starting within 48 hours of symptom onset, unless there is an allergy to antiplatelet therapy or active bleeding. Recommended therapy consists of aspirin 160-325 mg once daily, clopidogrel 75 mg once daily, or combination low-dose aspirin 25 mg plus extended-release dipyridamole 200 mg twice daily. Based on results from the International Stroke Trial (IST) and the Chinese Acute Stroke Trial (CAST) (pp. 117-118), it has been estimated that for every 1000 acute strokes treated with early aspirin therapy, 9 deaths or nonfatal strokes are prevented in the first few weeks and 13 fewer patients will be dead or dependent at 6 months.

B. Heparin Therapy
   1. Clinical Trials. The use of heparin for acute ischemic stroke is controversial. In small studies, heparin has been of benefit in the setting of cardiac embolism (Stroke 1983;14:668), but not for

progressing stroke or crescendo TIAs. Two larger studies—one using subcutaneous heparin (IST, p. 118) and another using a synthetic IV heparinoid (TOAST, p. 119)—failed to demonstrate a benefit for early anticoagulation. However, efficacy was not evaluated by stroke mechanism in IST, and subgroups may not have been large enough to demonstrate benefit for a given stroke mechanism in TOAST.

2. **Recommendations.** Given the high risk of stroke progression or recurrence, and until more data are available, it is reasonable to administer IV heparin acutely to lytic-ineligible patients with ischemic stroke if vascular imaging or echocardiography identifies a cardiac source of embolism or recent atherothrombosis of a large extracranial or intracranial artery. Heparin should also be considered for patients in whom a cardiac source of embolism or high-grade or complete large artery stenosis/occlusion is suspected clinically until vascular imaging and echocardiography are performed. A large brain infarct is a relative contraindication to heparin use.

3. **Heparin Dose.** Unfractionated heparin should be given as an IV infusion (without bolus) starting at 800-1000 U/hr and adjusted to maintain the PTT at 1.5-2.5 times control. Heparin is usually continued until the mechanism of stroke is identified and more definitive treatment is instituted. Low-molecular-weight heparin reduced mortality in one randomized trial (p. 118) but is not yet approved for use in stroke in the U.S.

Measures to Prevent Recurrent Stroke

Following acute therapy with tPA or aspirin/heparin (lytic-ineligible patients), therapeutic measures are indicated to reduce the risk of recurrent ischemic stroke. For ischemic stroke caused by large artery atherothrombosis, preventive measures depend on the culprit vessel and stenosis severity (Table 2.2). For ischemic stroke caused by brain embolism, preventive measures depend on the source of embolism (Table 2.3).

Table 2.2. Therapeutic Measures To Prevent Recurrent Ischemic Stroke Due To Large Artery Atherothrombosis[†]

Internal Carotid Artery		
Stenosis	**Therapy**	**Comments**
Total occlusion (100%)	Short-term heparin (PTT 1.5-2.5 x control) followed by warfarin (INR 2.0-3.0) x 6 weeks	Maintain blood pressure and volume status. Anticoagulant therapy may prevent clot propagation and embolization of fresh clot.
Severe stenosis (70-99%)	Urgent CEA[‡]. Otherwise, treat with long-term warfarin	If the deficit is stable, revascularization may be deferred for 3-6 weeks to decrease the risk of intracerebral hemorrhage associated with early carotid surgery. CEA reduces stroke rate and improves survival.
Plaque disease (50-69%)	Men: CEA[‡] plus antiplatelet therapy.* Women: antiplatelet therapy*	NASCET II (p. 123) trial demonstrated benefit of CEA in men with symptomatic 50-70% carotid stenosis. Antiplatelet therapy reduces vascular events by 20% following TIA or mild stroke (pp. 114-116).
Stenosis < 50%	Antiplatelet therapy.* Also consider omega-3 oils (1 gm tid)	

CEA = carotid endarterectomy
† Therapeutic measures following acute reperfusion therapy with tPA or acute antithrombotic therapy with aspirin or heparin (see pp. 16-17). Cardiovascular and cerebrovascular risk reduction measures are required for all patients (Chapters 8-13).
* Aspirin (325 mg/d), clopidogrel (75 mg/d), or combination low-dose aspirin plus extended-release dipyridamole (25mg/200mg bid). Consider combination aspirin (81-325 mg/d) plus clopidogrel (75 mg/d) for high-risk patients, especially those at increased risk of cardiac events. See discussion, pp. 77-85. For plaque disease some studies suggest benefit with lower-dose aspirin (81-165 mg/d).
‡ Carotid stenting may be considered for high-risk patients.

Table 2.2.   Therapeutic Measures To Prevent Recurrent Ischemic Stroke Due To Large Artery Atherothrombosis[†] (cont'd)

Vertebral Artery		
Severity	**Therapy**	**Comments**
Total occlusion (100%)	Short-term heparin (PTT 1.5-2.5 x control) followed by warfarin (INR 2.0-3.0) x 3-6 weeks	Maintain blood pressure and volume status. Anticoagulation may prevent clot propagation and embolization of fresh clot.
Severe stenosis (70-99%)	Long-term warfarin. Surgery and balloon angioplasty/stenting have been successfully performed	Monitor stenosis noninvasively every 6 months. If total occlusion develops, continue anticoagulation for an additional 3-6 weeks to prevent propagation of clot in-situ.
Plaque disease (< 70%)	Antiplatelet therapy*	For symptomatic TIAs or mild stroke, platelet inhibitors may be more effective at reducing stroke and death in the vertebrobasilar circulation than in the carotid circulation (Lancet 1987;2:1351).

[†]   Therapeutic measures following acute reperfusion therapy with tPA or acute antithrombotic therapy with aspirin or heparin (see pp. 16-17). Cardiovascular and cerebrovascular risk reduction measures are required for all patients (Chapters 8-13).

*   Aspirin (325 mg/d), clopidogrel (75 mg/d), or combination low-dose aspirin plus extended-release dipyridamole (25mg/200mg bid). Consider combination aspirin (81-325 mg/d) plus clopidogrel (75 mg/d) for high-risk patients, especially those at increased risk of cardiac events. See discussion, pp. 77-85. For plaque disease some studies suggest benefit with lower-dose aspirin (81-165 mg/d).

Table 2.2. Therapeutic Measures To Prevent Recurrent Ischemic Stroke Due To Large Artery Atherothrombosis† (cont'd)

Intracranial Disease		
Severity	**Therapy**	**Comments**
Total occlusion (100%)	Short-term warfarin (INR 2.0-3.0) x 3-6 weeks	Clinical manifestations depend on the culprit vessel (Figure 2.2): Anterior cerebral artery: contralateral sensorimotor loss (leg > arm/face). Posterior cerebral artery: hemianopia ± hemisensory loss.
Severe stenosis (50-99%)	Long-term warfarin (INR 2.0-3.0) while monitoring stenosis severity with ultrasound/MRA. If total occlusion develops, continue anticoagulation for an additional 3 weeks to prevent propagation of clot in-situ	Basilar artery: bilateral weakness, cranial nerve paralysis. The benefit of warfarin compared to aspirin for symptomatic intracranial disease (stenosis 50-99%) is supported by one retrospective trial showing a 46% reduction in major vascular events in patients treated with warfarin (Neurology 1995;45:1488). A prospective trial is underway.
Plaque disease (< 50%)	Antiplatelet therapy*	

† Therapeutic measures following acute reperfusion therapy with tPA or acute antithrombotic therapy with aspirin or heparin (see pp. 16-17). Cardiovascular and cerebrovascular risk reduction measures are required for all patients (Chapters 8-13).

* Aspirin (325 mg/d), clopidogrel (75 mg/d), or combination low-dose aspirin plus extended-release dipyridamole (25mg/200mg bid). Consider combination aspirin (81-325 mg/d) plus clopidogrel (75 mg/d) for high-risk patients, especially those at increased risk of cardiovascular events. See discussion, pp. 77-85. For plaque disease, some studies suggest benefit with lower-dose aspirin (81-165 mg/d).

Table 2.3. Therapeutic Measures To Prevent Recurrent Ischemic Stroke Due To Brain Embolism*

Source	Therapy	Comments
Atrial fibrillation (AF)	• For acute embolism, consider IV tPA or intraarterial thrombolysis with tPA or urokinase (experimental), depending on the presence/location of occlusive embolus • For primary and secondary prevention, treat with warfarin (INR 2.0-3.0) as long as AF persists. Aspirin or another antiplatelet agent may be considered for primary prevention of embolic stroke in patients < 60 years old with "lone" AF (i.e., no history of hypertension, heart disease, or prior embolism)	Incidence of systemic embolization is 5-6% per year, and most embolic events are cerebral. Warfarin reduces stroke by 50-80% and improves survival in nonvalvular AF (pp. 111-113). Hemorrhagic transformation occurs in 20-30% of embolic strokes; therefore, some initiate anticoagulation only if a CT/MRI at day 3-5 is negative for hemorrhage, especially if the area of infarction is large. Even if hemorrhagic transformation occurs, it is usually well-tolerated (exception: symptomatic hemorrhage with tPA). Ximelagatran, an oral thrombin inhibitor, was a safe/effective alternative to warfarin in SPORTIF-III (p. 113).
Acute myocardial infarction (MI)	For primary prevention of stroke, consider warfarin (INR 2.0-3.0) x 3-6 months for acute MI complicated by ventricular aneurysm, mural thrombus (especially if large or pedunculated), or a large area of hypokinesis	The incidence of systemic embolization following anterior MI and inferior MI is 6% and 1%, respectively, and most embolic events are cerebral. The risk of embolization is highest for protruding LV thrombus, especially in the first few months after MI. Acute stroke during thrombolytic therapy for acute MI is often hemorrhagic and may require drainage of hematoma.

Table 2.3. Therapeutic Measures To Prevent Recurrent Ischemic Stroke Due To Brain Embolism*

Source	Therapy	Comments
Valvular heart disease	• For primary prevention of stroke, no specific therapy is recommended for native valve disease with sinus rhythm. For prosthetic valves, treat with warfarin (INR 3.0-4.5) long term. • For prevention of recurrent stroke, treat with warfarin for native valve disease (INR 2.0-3.0) and prosthetic valves (INR 3.0-4.5). For embolization despite warfarin, options include intensification of warfarin therapy, addition of low-dose aspirin (81-165 mg/d) or possibly other antiplatelets, or valve surgery	The risk of embolization in patients with rheumatic mitral stenosis and AF is increased 17-fold compared to patients without valve disease in sinus rhythm. Embolization rates for mechanical mitral valves, mechanical aortic valves, and bioprosthetic valves are 4%, 2%, and 1% per year, respectively.
Cardio-myopathy	In a retrospective trial of patients with ejection fractions < 20% and heart failure, warfarin decreased the rate of cardiac embolization compared to aspirin (J Am Coll Cardiol 1993;21:218A). Prospective trials are needed to confirm this finding	The source of emboli is usually LV mural thrombus, which develops as a result of poor systolic function and blood stasis.
Atrial myxoma	Surgical excision is indicated for the prevention of recurrent stroke	Atrial myxoma is the most common primary cardiac tumor and can mimic mitral valve disease (stenosis/regurgitation) or infectious endocarditis.

Table 2.3. Therapeutic Measures To Prevent Recurrent Ischemic Stroke Due To Brain Embolism*

Source	Therapy	Comments
Paradoxical embolism	For prevention of recurrent stroke, warfarin is indicated if the patient has a proven venous clot until the atrial septal defect (ASD) is repaired	ASD and patent foramen ovale are the most common routes for paradoxical embolus. Contrast echo with Valsalva maneuver, which can visualize interatrial communications, is recommended for all young patients with unexplained stroke. Paradoxical embolism can also occur in older age groups.
Other cardiac conditions	• Aspirin (325 mg/d) is indicated for the prevention of recurrent embolic stroke due to mitral valve prolapse, mitral annular calcification, calcified aortic valve, marantic endocarditis. For recurrences on aspirin, treat with warfarin long term • For emboli due to infectious endocarditis, treat with antibiotics. Anticoagulation does not prevent embolization and increases the risk of bleeding from a mycotic aneurysm or cerebral embolus	Marantic (non-bacterial thrombotic [NBTE]) endocarditis is a common cause of stroke in patients with cancer or other chronic debilitating illnesses. Marantic vegetations and vegetations in patients with systemic lupus erythematosus or antiphospholipid antibody syndrome consist of friable platelet-fibrin nodules, usually along the valve commissures. A single embolus is not an indication for valve surgery in infectious endocarditis, but valve replacement should be considered for recurrent emboli despite appropriate antimicrobial therapy. Embolization rate after 24 hours of antibiotic control is low (< 5%).

* Cardiovascular and cerebrovascular risk reduction measures are required for all patients (Chapters 8-13)

Lacunar Stroke

Lacunar stroke accounts for 15-20% of ischemic strokes and is caused by atherothrombotic or lipohyalinotic occlusion of one of the small penetrating branches of the circle of Willis, middle cerebral artery, or vertebral/basilar arteries. Occlusion results in a small infarct of the deep brain structures (basal ganglia, cerebral white matter, thalamus, pons, cerebellum), ranging in size from 3 mm to 2 cm. Risk factors include hypertension, diabetes, and polycythemia. The neurological deficit of lacunar infarction is typically fluctuating, stepwise progressive, or remitting, and gradually worsens over days. Patients are usually alert without headache or vomiting. Lacunar stroke is preceded by TIAs in 25% of cases and presents as one of several well-defined syndromes, including: pure motor hemiparesis (contralateral hemiparesis; dysarthria; no sensory or visual loss or cognitive impairment); pure sensory stroke (contralateral sensory loss or paresthesias; no motor loss, dysarthria, visual loss, or cognitive impairment); dysarthria-clumsy-hand syndrome (dysarthria; dysphagia; weakness of contralateral face and tongue; paresis and clumsiness of contralateral arm and hand); ataxic hemiparesis (prominent ataxia of contralateral leg and arm; paresis of contralateral leg and side of face); isolated motor/sensory stroke (paresis or sensory loss of contralateral leg, arm, or face; no visual loss or cognitive impairment). Management includes long-term control of blood pressure and empiric antiplatelet therapy. Omega-3 oils (1 gm tid) can be used to decrease whole blood viscosity and possibly improve blood flow through narrowed penetrating arteries. Some experts argue that lacunar stroke should not be treated with thrombolytics; however, patients with lacunes were included in the NINDS tPA trial (p. 121). Prognosis is good for recovery of function, although other lacunes frequently develop.

Transient Ischemic Attack

Transient ischemic attacks are brief episodes of neurological dysfunction caused by reversible ischemia in a vascular territory. The term "TIA" is used to encompass episodes lasting less than 24 hours; however, most TIAs last less than one hour, and the majority of vascular neurological symptoms persisting for more than one hour are unlikely to fully resolve. Patients with transient symptoms often develop ischemic lesions on brain imaging, blurring the distinction between TIA and stroke. The mechanisms, work-up, and treatment of TIA are the same as for ischemic stroke.

Chapter 3

Thrombolytic Therapy for Acute Ischemic Stroke

A. **Overview.** The rationale for thrombolytic therapy, which activates plasminogen to degrade thrombus via breakdown of fibrin (Figure 3.1), is based on studies demonstrating that 80% of ischemic strokes are caused by occlusive clot and that neuronal death and brain infarction are time-dependent events (Stroke 2003;34:1056-83). When used in strict accordance with the National Institute of Neurological Diseases and Stroke (NINDS) tPA study protocol, IV administration of tPA within 3 hours of stroke onset increases the likelihood of minimal or no disability by 30% or more. To be maximally effective, tPA should be administered within 3 hours of symptom onset; late administration has not been shown to be effective and increases the risk of intracerebral hemorrhage. Although not approved for this indication, some neurologists administer tPA to carefully selected patients between 3-6 hours after stroke onset if a diffusion/perfusion MRI demonstrates vascular occlusion with no or minor brain infarction and a large area of brain tissue that is underperfused but not yet infarcted. Such selection must be highly individualized due to the increased risk of brain hemorrhage when tPA is administered late. For patients presenting with middle cerebral artery infarction within 6 hours of stroke onset, intraarterial thrombolysis using pro-urokinase has been shown to improve outcome at 90 days in the PROACT II trial (p. 121). Because pro-urokinase is not available in the U.S., intraarterial tPA is being used in a similar fashion at select sites with interventional neuroradiological capability. Intraarterial thrombolysis may improve recanalization rates, but time delay to onset of therapy has been an important limitation of this approach. Newer thrombolytic and antiplatelet agents have been used in small series of

patients, including retaplase (Neurosurgery 2001;49:41-50), abciximab
(Stroke 2000;31:601-609; AbESST trial, p. 117), and the combination
of abciximab or integrelin with tPA or retaplase (Neurology
2001;56:1585-87; Stroke 2002;33:359). Thrombectomy, laser,
ultrasound devices, and balloon angioplasty/stenting in conjunction with
antiplatelet, antithrombin, and thrombolytic therapy is under
investigation. Thrombolytic therapy represents a major advance in the
treatment of acute ischemic stroke but is now only applicable to 2-5% of
patients, primarily due to delays in hospital presentation. Efforts to teach
individuals to recognize the symptoms of stroke and the need to seek
immediate medical attention will increase the utilization of thrombolytic
therapy. Secondary prevention measures can reduce the risk of recurrent
stroke by 25-50% and are mandatory for all patients (Chapters 8-13).

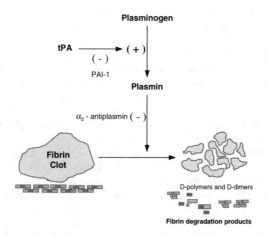

Figure 3.1. Thrombolytic Therapy and Dissolution of Clot

tPA = tissue plasminogen activator, PAI-1 = plasminogen activator inhibitor.
Thrombolytic agents activate plasminogen, which degrades thrombus via breakdown
of fibrin. Fibrin breakdown results in the release of fibrin degradation products (D-
dimers and other D-polymers).

B. Baseline Evaluation. Inclusion and exclusion criteria for thrombolytic therapy are shown in Table 3.1. Ideal candidates present within 3 hours of stroke onset and have no hemorrhage on CT scan and NIH stroke scores of 4-20 (i.e., moderate deficit) (Table 3.2). Patients with scores ≤ 4 (no or very mild deficit) have a very good prognosis and may not benefit from tPA, while patients with scores > 20 (severe deficit) are at increased risk of intracerebral hemorrhage; individualization of therapy based on an estimate of the risk/benefit ratio is required in these cases. Baseline laboratory evaluation in lytic-eligible patients includes fibrinogen, hemoglobin, hematocrit, PT/PTT, and platelet count; type and cross 4 units packed red blood cells is also recommended.

C. Dosing and Administration of Thrombolytic Therapy. tPA is given at a total dose of 0.9 mg/kg (maximum 90 mg): 10% of the total dose is given as an IV bolus over 1 minute, and the remaining 90% is administered as a constant IV infusion over 60 minutes. Anticoagulants and antiplatelets are withheld for the next 24 hours. For suspected cardiogenic embolism or large vessel atherothrombosis, heparin is often started 24 hours after lytic therapy as an IV infusion (without bolus) of 800-1000 U/hr and adjusted to a PTT of 1.5-2.5 times control until the diagnostic evaluation is complete and definitive therapy is instituted. Antihypertensive therapy is administered as needed to maintain blood pressure < 180/105 mmHg.

D. Post-Lytic Care
   1. **General Measures.** Following thrombolytic therapy, vital signs and neurological status should be checked every 15 minutes for the first 2 hours, every 30 minutes x 6 hours, then hourly x 18 hours. To minimize the risk of intracerebral hemorrhage, blood pressure should be maintained < 180/105 mmHg and antiplatelet and anticoagulant therapy should be withheld for 24 hours. Blood draws and invasive lines/procedures should also be avoided for 24 hours after thrombolysis, if possible.

**Table 3.1. Thrombolytic Therapy for Acute Ischemic Stroke:
Inclusion and Exclusion Criteria**

Inclusion Criteria
- Stroke onset < 3 hours. Time of onset is the time when the patient was last known to be normal. If time of onset is uncertain, tPA should not be given, with the possible exception that diffusion/perfusion MRI and MRA show a vascular occlusion with no or minor brain infarction and a large area of brain tissue that is underperfused but not yet infarcted. tPA is approved only for IV administration within 3 hours of stroke onset
- No hemorrhage on CT scan
- Early infarct not > 1/3 of middle cerebral artery territory
- Screening NIH stroke score (Table 3.2). Ideal candidates for thrombolytic therapy have scores of 4-20 (mild to moderate deficit). Patients with scores ≤ 4 (no or very mild deficit) have a very good prognosis and may not benefit from tPA. Patients with scores > 20 (severe deficit) are at increased risk of intracerebral hemorrhage; individualized therapy based on an estimate of the risk/benefit ratio is required in these cases

Exclusion Criteria
- Active bleeding
- Systolic BP > 185 mmHg or diastolic BP > 110 mmHg
- Aggressive treatment required to reduce blood pressure to specified limits
- Rapidly improving or minor symptoms
- Seizure at onset of stroke
- Symptoms of subarachnoid hemorrhage
- Prior intracerebral hemorrhage felt by examiner to predispose patient to high risk of recurrence
- Stroke or head trauma within 3 months
- Myocardial infarction within 3 months
- Major surgery or other serious trauma within 2 weeks
- Gastrointestinal or urinary tract hemorrhage within 21 days
- Arterial puncture at a noncompressible site within 7 days
- Taking anticoagulants or receiving heparin within 48 hours
- INR > 1.5 or elevated PTT
- Platelet count < 100,000/mm^3
- Glucose < 50 mg/dL or > 400 mg/dL
- Pregnancy or lactation

2. **Management of Elevated Blood Pressure**
    a. **Systolic blood pressure > 180 mmHg or diastolic blood pressure > 105 mmHg** on two consecutive readings 5-10 minutes apart. Consider treatment with labetalol 10 mg IV over 1-2 minutes. The dose can be repeated or doubled every 10-20 minutes up to a total cumulative dose of 300 mg. If a satisfactory response is not obtained, nitroprusside can be administered at a dose of 0.5-10 mcg/kg/min. Blood pressure should be monitored every 10 minutes during IV therapy and the patient observed for hypotension. (If systolic blood pressure > 230 mmHg or diastolic blood pressure 121-140 mmHg and labetalol is contraindicated, consider enalapril 1.25-2.5 mg IV every 6 hours.)
    b. **Diastolic blood pressure > 140 mmHg.** Treatment with IV sodium nitroprusside at 0.5-10 mcg/kg/minute is recommended. Blood pressure should be monitored every 10 minutes during IV therapy and the patient observed for hypotension.

E. **Management of Lytic Complications.** If acute deterioration in neurologic status develops during tPA infusion, intracerebral hemorrhage should be suspected. In this situation it is important to immediately discontinue the tPA infusion and obtain an emergency unenhanced head CT to confirm the diagnosis. For life-threatening hemorrhage, urgent treatment includes transfusion of 6-8 units of platelets and 4-6 units of cryoprecipitate. Aminocaproic acid should also be given at a dose of 4-5 gm IV over 1 hour followed by 1 gm PO or IV push hourly until bleeding is controlled. Fibrinogen levels should be rechecked every 4 hours and cryoprecipitate transfused as needed to maintain fibrinogen levels > 150 mg/dL. Periodic CBC and PT/PTT measurements should also be obtained. If blood transfusion is required, the patient should be typed and crossmatched for 4 units of packed red blood cells, 4-6 units of cryoprecipitate or fresh frozen plasma, and 1 unit of single-donor platelets.

Table 3.2. National Institutes of Health Stroke Scale (maximum = 42)

Response	(Score)	Response	(Score)
Level of consciousness		Motor arm (left and right)	
alert	(0)	no drift	(0)
drowsy	(1)	drift before 10 seconds	(1)
stuporous	(2)	falls before 10 seconds	(2)
coma	(3)	no effort against gravity	(3)
		no movement	(4)
Response to level of consciousness questions*		Motor leg (left and right)	
answers both correctly	(0)	no drift	(0)
answers one correctly	(1)	drift before 5-10 seconds	(1)
answers neither correctly	(2)	falls before 5-10 seconds	(2)
		no effort against gravity	(3)
		no movement	(4)
Response to level of consciousness commands†		Ataxia	
obeys both correctly	(0)	absent	(0)
obeys one correctly	(1)	one limb	(1)
obeys neither	(2)	two limbs	(2)
Pupillary response		Sensory	
both reactive	(0)	normal	(0)
one reactive	(1)	mild	(1)
neither reactive	(2)	severe loss	(2)
Gaze		Language	
normal	(0)	normal	(0)
partial gaze palsy	(1)	mild aphasia	(1)
total gaze palsy	(2)	severe aphasia	(2)
		mute or global aphasia	(3)
Visual fields		Facial palsy	
no visual loss	(0)	normal	(0)
partial hemianopsia	(1)	minor paralysis	(1)
complete hemianopsia	(2)	partial paralysis	(2)
bilateral hemianopsia	(3)	complete paralysis	(3)
Dysarthria		Extinction/inattention	
normal	(0)	normal	(0)
mild	(1)	mild	(1)
severe	(2)	severe	(2)

* Level of consciousness questions: "How old are you?" "What month is this?"
† Level of consciousness commands: "Squeeze my hand" (using nonparetic hand), "Close your eyes."

Chapter 4
Brain Hemorrhage

Hemorrhagic stroke can be readily classified into subarachnoid hemorrhage, intracerebral hemorrhage, and subdural/extradural hemorrhage based on clinical presentation and CT scan (Table 4.1).

- **Subarachnoid hemorrhage** presents with sudden onset severe headache, cessation of activities, and vomiting without focal neurologic signs. CT scan shows blood in the subarachnoid space and brain cisterns, and spinal fluid is always bloody.

- **Intracerebral hemorrhage** presents with focal neurologic symptoms. Headache, vomiting, and decreased consciousness often accompany larger hemorrhages. CT and MRI show a hematoma within the brain.

- **Subdural and extradural hemorrhage** are usually caused by head trauma. Lesions are outside the brain, either inside (subdural) or outside (extradural) the dura mater.

Depending on the type and cause of brain hemorrhage, management includes prevention of rebleeding and vasospasm; correction of bleeding diatheses; control of hypertension; lowering of increased intracranial pressure; surgical clipping, ligation, or coating of ruptured aneurysms; excision of AV malformations and cavernous angiomas; and drainage of hematomas.

Table 4.1. Hemorrhagic Stroke: Clinical Features

	Subarachnoid Hemorrhage	Intracerebral Hemorrhage	Subdural/Epidural Hematoma
Risk factors	Hypertension, bleeding disorders, drugs, trauma. Often occurs in absence of risk factors	Hypertension, bleeding disorders, amyloid angiopathy, drugs (amphetamines, cocaine), trauma	Old age, falls, head injury, anticoagulants
Onset of neurological deficit	Sudden, typically during exertion. Warning leak occurs in 15-30% as a headache ("sentinel headache") that often goes unrecognized. Focal neurologic signs may be absent or manifest as subtle hemiparesis or oculomotor nerve palsies	Symptoms gradually progress over minutes to hours. Occasional onset with exertion or stress. Focal neurologic deficit is prominent and suggests location of hemorrhage	Gradual (usually slight) weakness and numbness on one side
Associated symptoms	Sudden onset of severe headache, cessation of activity, vomiting, nuchal rigidity. Initial loss of consciousness, seizures, confusion, agitation, photophobia ± phonophobia	Headache, vomiting, decreased consciousness, seizures, especially with large bleed. Headache is absent in 50%, especially with smaller bleed	Headache, diminished alertness
Stroke location	Subarachnoid, occasionally meningocerebral	Deep brain structures (basal ganglia, cerebral white matter, thalamus, pons, cerebellum)	Extracerebral blood
Imaging	CT: hyperdensity (bright) MRI: dark (T1-weighted images); bright (T2-weighted images). Location in subarachnoid space. MRI may be less sensitive for detection of subarachnoid blood than CT scan	CT: focal hyperdensity (bright) MRI: acute (< 24 hrs) (dark on T1 images; bright on T2 images); subacute (1-5 days) (dark on T1/T2 images); chronic (months) (bright on T1/T2 images). Location within brain parenchyma, often spreading to surface and/or ventricles. Dark on T2 star-weighted images	CT: hyperdensity (bright) over convexity of brain MRI: abnormal signal in subdural/epidural space

Table 4.1. Hemorrhagic Stroke: Clinical Features

	Subarachnoid Hemorrhage	Intracerebral Hemorrhage	Subdural/Epidural Hematoma
Treatment	Clipping or coiling of berry aneurysms (early) and AV malformations (late). Prevention of rebleeding/vasospasm; control of intracranial pressure	Control of hypertension, increased intracranial pressure, bleeding diathesis. Surgical drainage of large putaminal, lobar, cerebellar hematomas	Surgical drainage if large
Prognosis	<u>Ruptured aneurysm:</u> High morbidity and mortality. Early re-bleed with vasospasm and cerebral infarction are common. Overall, 33% of patients die before reaching the hospital, 20% die in the hospital or have severe disability, 17% deteriorate in the hospital, and only 30% do well. Rebleed rate is 3% per year in patients without surgery <u>Ruptured AV malformation:</u> Better prognosis than after ruptured aneurysm. Early rebleed/vasospasm uncommon. Mortality with first hemorrhage is 10%. Rebleed rate is 0.5-2% per year with 20% mortality	Size of bleed determines outcome. One month mortality is 30%. The probability of significant functional recovery is greater following intracerebral hemorrhage (tissue is pushed aside) than following cerebral infarction (tissue is rendered necrotic due to ischemia)	Excellent if drained before brain herniation

Subarachnoid Hemorrhage

A. **Ruptured Saccular (Berry) Aneurysm**

 1. **Overview.** Ruptured berry aneurysms are responsible for 80% of subarachnoid hemorrhages. The vast majority (> 90%) of berry aneurysms originate from the anterior circle of Willis, and those that rupture are usually > 5 mm in diameter. Patients are usually asymptomatic prior to rupture, although 15-30% have a warning leak, manifest as a headache ("sentinel headache") that often goes unrecognized. The onset of neurological deficit—severe headache, cessation of activity, vomiting, stiff neck—is sudden and typically occurs during exertion. Most patients present without focal neurologic deficit, although a third-nerve palsy (PCOM aneurysm), hemiparesis and aphasia (MCA aneurysm), or paraparesis and encephalopathy (ACA aneurysm) may occur. Patients can also awaken with headache, confusion, stiff neck, and high fever. Conditions associated with berry aneurysm include coarctation of the aorta, fibromuscular dysplasia, polycystic kidney disease, Marfan's syndrome, Ehlers-Danlos, hereditary hemorrhagic telangectasia, neurofibromatosis, and pseudoxanthoma elasticum. Hypertension, bleeding disorders, and trauma increase the risk of subarachnoid hemorrhage, but subarachnoid hemorrhage often occurs in the absence of risk factors. The diagnosis of ruptured aneurysm is made by CT scan, which is 85-90% sensitive. If a CT scan is negative and the index of suspicion is high, a lumbar puncture should be performed; a normal lumbar puncture excludes the diagnosis of subarachnoid hemorrhage. Angiography may at first fail to identify the site of bleeding because of vasospasm. In these cases, angiography should be repeated at 2 weeks. Morbidity and mortality rates are high, and early rebleeding and vasospasm with cerebral infarction are common. Overall, 33% of patients die before reaching the hospital, 20% die in the hospital or have significant disability, 17% deteriorate in the hospital, and only 30% do well. Rebleeding occurs in 3% of patients without surgery.

2. **Treatment.** Treatment of subarachnoid hemorrhage includes bed rest in a dark, quiet setting, gentle hydration, and prophylactic anticonvulsant therapy (e.g., phenytoin 300-400 mg/d in divided doses to maintain plasma levels at 10-20 mcg/mL). Four-vessel angiography is recommended in all patients, and surgical clipping, coiling, or ligation is performed to reduce rebleeding and improve survival. A recent trial (ISAT, p. 126) found that patients treated with endovascular coils had improved outcomes compared to clipping. Embolization or coiling of ruptured aneurysms may be indicated when the aneurysm is relatively inaccessible (e.g., basilar) or the patient is a poor operative risk. Surgery is warranted as soon as possible (within 72 hours) for patients who are alert, oriented, and have no focal deficit (Hunt and Hess Class I or II) (J Neurosurg 1968;28:14). For the remaining patients, surgical intervention is performed at 10-14 days. Nimodipine is recommended to reduce vasospasm, which complicates 25-35% of subarachnoid hemorrhages and often results in cerebral infarction. The dose of nimodipine is 60 mg (PO) every 4 hours x 21 days (Br Med J 1989;298:636).

B. **Ruptured AV Malformation**
   1. **Overview.** Ruptured AV malformations account for 10% of subarachnoid hemorrhages. AV malformations typically present as subarachnoid hemorrhage (45%), seizures (35%), or progressive neurologic deficit (20%); chronic, migraine-like headaches may occur in some. Pregnant females with AV malformations are at increased risk of subarachnoid hemorrhage, especially during the first trimester of pregnancy and during labor. The diagnosis of ruptured AV malformation is made by MRA and angiography. Prognosis is better than for ruptured aneurysm; mortality rates are 10% with the first bleed and 20% with a second bleed. Early vasospasm and rebleeding are uncommon, and the rate of rebleeding is 0.5-2% per year.
   2. **Treatment.** Younger patients in good condition are treated by delayed surgical excision. Adjunctive embolization may also be considered in certain cases. For elderly patients and those with severe neurologic deficit, radiation therapy or embolization may be appropriate. Patients with seizures without subarachnoid hemorrhage

are treated with anticonvulsant therapy without surgery.

C. Complications of Subarachnoid Hemorrhage

1. **Rebleeding.** Without early surgical treatment, many ruptured berry aneurysms rebleed—20% within 2 weeks, 30% within 1 month, 40% within 6 months—and rebleeding is associated with a mortality rate of 40%. Rebleeding typically presents as sudden severe headache, meningismus, and rapid development of coma; focal neurologic signs indicate the presence of intraparenchymal hemorrhage or vasospasm. Prevention is the key to therapy: adequate analgesia, control of hypertension, sedation, laxatives, and early surgery reduce the risk of rebleeding. In contrast to berry aneurysms, acute rebleeding is uncommon after ruptured AV malformation.

2. **Vasospasm.** Symptomatic vasospasm complicates 25-35% of ruptured berry aneurysms, usually between days 4-14, and most episodes result in cerebral infarction. Vasospasm typically presents as decreased level of alertness with or without hypertension and ECG changes; focal neurologic signs may also be present. Treatment consists of hypervolemic hemodilution (3 liters of fluid per day) to decrease blood viscosity and maintain cerebral blood flow. Early (within 10 days) administration of the calcium antagonist nimodipine reduces the risk of death or dependency within 3 months of aneurysmal subarachnoid hemorrhage by 24% (Neurology 1998;50:876-83). The dose of nimodipine is 60 mg (PO) q4h x 21 days.

3. **Increased intracranial pressure** (see pp. 40-41).

4. **Hydrocephalus.** Hydrocephalus can be acute or subacute (2-4 weeks) and manifests as increasing headache, lethargy, incontinence, and decreased spontaneity. The diagnosis is confirmed by CT scan or MRI. Treatment consists of surgical (ventricular) drainage or repeat lumbar punctures.

5. **Intracerebral hematoma.** Surgical evacuation is often performed for hematomas resulting in mass effect.

6. **Cardiac.** ECG abnormalities occur in more than 50% of patients after subarachnoid hemorrhage and can persist for days. ECG changes can mimic acute myocardial infarction/ischemia and include long QT interval, ST segment elevation or depression, giant upright

or inverted T waves, and prominent U waves. Arrhythmias are common following subarachnoid hemorrhage and include sinus tachycardia, sinus bradycardia, tachy-brady syndrome, wandering atrial pacemaker, and AV junctional rhythm. Ventricular tachycardia occurs infrequently.

7. **Hyponatremia.** Hyponatremia may be due to the syndrome of inappropriate ADH and is associated with a poor prognosis.

Intracerebral Hemorrhage

Intracerebral hemorrhage usually results from an acute rise in blood pressure and primarily involves the deep brain structures, including the basal ganglia, cerebral white matter, thalamus, pons, and cerebellum. Other causes of intracranial hemorrhage include bleeding disorders, amyloid angiopathy, drugs (amphetamines, cocaine), and trauma. Most patients present with a focal neurological deficit, which suggests the location of hemorrhage, and symptoms gradually progress over minutes to hours. Large bleeds are accompanied by headaches, vomiting, decreased consciousness, and seizures. In contrast, headache may be absent in 50% of smaller bleeds. On CT scan, intracerebral hemorrhage presents as a focal hyperdensity (bright); on MRI, acute hematomas are dark and chronic hematomas are white on T1- and T2-weighted images. Treatment consists of control of hypertension and increased intracranial pressure, correction of bleeding diatheses, and surgical drainage of large putaminal, lobar, or cerebellar hematomas. Prognosis depends on the size of the bleed. Overall, 1-month mortality is 30%. The probability of significant functional recovery is greater following intracerebral hemorrhage than following cerebral infarction, as brain tissue is more likely to be pushed aside (bleed) than rendered necrotic (ischemic infarction).

A. **Hypertension.** Many intracerebral bleeds result from an acute rise in blood pressure, which causes rupture of a normal or microaneurysmal or lipohyalinotic segment of a small resistance artery. Elderly patients are at increased risk and can develop hemorrhage at lower blood pressures than younger individuals. Papilledema may lag behind clinical improvement and is not necessarily a sign of worsening. Rebleeding at the same site does not usually occur. The goal of therapy is to lower systolic blood pressure to ≤ 160 mmHg (10-20% reduction over the first hour followed by more gradual reduction over the next 12-24 hours). Nitroprusside or labetalol are often used for this purpose. Since the acute phase of stroke is associated with impaired cerebral autoregulation, marked reductions in blood pressure may induce cerebral hypoperfusion. Therefore, if neurologic function deteriorates during antihypertensive therapy, drug dosage should be reduced or discontinued. In addition to blood pressure control, it is important to reduce elevated intracranial pressure and to surgically drain large putaminal, lobar, or cerebellar hematomas.

B. Other Causes of Intracerebral Hemorrhage. In addition to an acute rise in blood pressure, intracerebral hemorrhage may occur as a result of ruptured AV malformation, amyloid angiopathy, bleeding diathesis, trauma, or hemorrhage into an infarct or tumor. Intracerebral hemorrhage caused by illicit drug use (amphetamines, cocaine) usually occurs within a few minutes of exposure and manifests as headache, confusion, and seizures; mortality rates are high (20-30%). Depending on the cause, treatment varies from surgical excision of AV malformations to reversal of bleeding diatheses. For intracerebral hemorrhage that develops during anticoagulation or thrombolytic therapy, restoration of normal clotting function is imperative. For patients receiving warfarin, the drug should be immediately discontinued and 2-3 units of fresh frozen plasma IV (or 5-25 mg vitamin K) should be administered. The PT should be checked in 6 hours and fresh frozen plasma transfused as needed to restore clotting function. For patients receiving heparin, the heparin infusion should be discontinued and protamine sulfate 20-30 mg (IV infusion) considered. For patients receiving a thrombolytic, the drug should be immediately discontinued and 6 units of cryoprecipitate given IV to increase the fibrinogen level to > 150 mg/dL. Fibrinogen levels should be rechecked in 4-6 hours and cryoprecipitate transfused as needed.

C. Cerebellar Hemorrhage. Ten percent of intracerebral hemorrhages occur within the cerebellum. Symptoms include inability to walk, vomiting, and headache; patients are usually alert at onset. Large bleeds often result in brainstem compression, which manifests as increasing stupor, lateral gaze palsy (toward hematoma), and a bilateral extensor plantar response. More than 75% of those awake at presentation progress to coma, which may be complicated by hypotension and respiratory depression. Surgical drainage is indicated for hemorrhage > 3 cm in diameter, especially when accompanied by decreased consciousness.

D. Subdural and Extradural Hematoma. Most subdural hematomas are caused by laceration of bridging or cortical veins as a result of head trauma. Depending on the acuity and size of the hematoma, symptoms range from rapid deterioration in mental status and alertness to gradual, subtle weakness and numbness on one side. The diagnosis is made by CT scan. Treatment consists of surgical drainage of large hematomas and reversal of coagulation abnormalities.

- *Acute subdural* hematomas usually occur after trauma or rapid deceleration. Mortality rates for patients with severe head injuries are high (40-50%), and many survivors will have permanent neurological deficits.

- *Subacute subdural* hematomas develop 2 days to 1 week after head injury and can also occur with chronic anticoagulant therapy. They are usually less severe than acute subdural hematomas, and the prognosis is good.

- *Chronic subdural* hematomas present with confusion, morning headache, unsteadiness and/or weakness 1-6 weeks after head injury, which may not be remembered by the patient. Bilateral hematomas are sometimes present.

- *Extradural hematomas* typically present with abrupt, persistent loss of consciousness. The classic history of transient loss of consciousness followed by a lucid interval and then rapid deterioration is uncommon. Extradural hematomas are often associated with skull fractures that tear the middle meningeal artery. Because the ruptured vessel is arterial (and thus under higher pressure), they can expand rapidly and lead to brain herniation and death. Correction of coagulation abnormalities and surgical evacuation is warranted.

Chapter 5

Stroke-Related Complications

Patients with stroke are at high risk for serious medical complications caused by atherosclerosis (myocardial ischemia/infarction), prolonged bed rest and immobility (decubitus ulcer, DVT, pulmonary embolism, depression, malnutrition), and as a direct consequence of the stroke itself (increased intracranial pressure, seizures, stress-induced GI ulcers, urinary voiding problems, aspiration pneumonia). Major bleeding complications can also occur from the use of anticoagulants and thrombolytics. The prevention and treatment of stroke-related complications are described in Table 5.1.

Table 5.1. Treatment of Stroke-Related Complications

Complication	Comments
Increased intracranial pressure (cont'd next page)	Increased intracranial pressure usually develops 1-4 days after stroke but may occur acutely within hours. Manifestations include headache, decreased consciousness, papilledema, contralateral hemisphere signs, and upper brainstem compression. The diagnosis is made by CT or MRI, which shows brain edema and a shift in intracranial contents. Aggressiveness of treatment depends on the severity, location, and potential reversibility of the culprit brain lesion. Therapeutic measures include: • Head of bed elevation. • Modest fluid restriction (2/3 of usual intake). Avoid hypotonic solutions (D_5W, 0.5 NS), which may increase cerebral edema. • Intubation/hyperventilation to induce hypocapnia (pCO_2 25-30 mmHg). Effects last 12-36 hours. Excessive lowering of pCO_2 may induce further ischemia. Opioids and benzodiazepines help patients tolerate prolonged bed rest and hyperventilatory support. Ketamine, high PEEP, volatile anesthetics, and tracheal suction can raise intracranial pressure. • Control of pain and agitation

Table 5.1. Treatment of Stroke-Related Complications

Complication	Comments
Increased intracranial pressure (cont'd)	• Osmotic agents (mannitol, glycerol) to increase serum osmolality to 300-310 mOsm. Mannitol is usually given as an initial dose of 0.5 gm/kg IV over 20 minutes, with repeat doses of 0.25 gm/kg q4-6h as needed up to a maximum cumulative dose of 2 gm/kg/d. The effect on intracranial pressure usually occurs in about 20 minutes. Fluids lost during osmotic diuresis should be replaced intravenously to prevent a hyperosmolor state and dehydration. A rebound increase in intracranial pressure may occur upon withdrawal. • High-dose barbiturates (e.g., thiopental 1-5 mg/kg) rapidly lower intracranial pressure but may cause respiratory/ myocardial depression and therefore require ventilatory support and blood pressure monitoring. • Drainage of CSF via intraventricular catheter for secondary hydrocephalus. • High-dose corticosteroids are useful for elevated intracranial pressure due to tumor, trauma, or abscess but not for anoxia or infarction. (Steroids may reduce extracellular vasogenic edema but are of little value for intracellular [cytotoxic] edema.) • Surgical decompression via removal/drainage of hematomas or infarcted temporal lobe/cerebellum. Hemicraniectomy can be performed to decompress intracranial pressure.
Seizures	Seizures complicate 5-20% of strokes. Most can be managed with phenytoin (18-20 mg/kg IV at a rate of 50 mg/min followed by 100 mg PO q8h to maintain blood levels of 10-20 mcg/mL). Benzodiazepines can be used to treat seizures acutely but increase the risk of respiratory depression and are not indicated for long-term control.
Deep venous thrombosis (DVT)	High incidence of DVT during recovery. Prevention is the key, with early ambulation, bedside physical therapy, and support hose or inflated stockings. To prevent DVT, unfractionated heparin (5,000 units SQ bid) or low-molecular-weight heparin (enoxaparin 0.5 mg/kg SQ q12h or 1.5 mg/kg q24h) should be administered in non-ambulatory patients in the absence of brain hemorrhage or other contraindications to anticoagulation.

Table 5.1. Treatment of Stroke-Related Complications

Complication	Comments
Pulmonary embolus (PE)	Treated with IV heparin unless recent brain hemorrhage. If multiple or life-threatening pulmonary emboli occur in the setting of recent brain hemorrhage, inferior venal caval umbrella or interruption is indicated. For large PE with hemodynamic compromise and no brain hemorrhage, thrombolytic therapy can be considered.
Depression	Depressive syndromes may be difficult to recognize in the stroke patient. Depression should be suspected if there is slower-than-expected recovery, poor cooperation in therapy, emotional lability, or flattened affect. Patients may respond well to traditional pharmacological therapy.
Hypertension	May be the cause or consequence of acute stroke. Blood pressure should not be treated in the acute stages of stroke unless > 200/120 mmHg (or > 180/105 mmHg after lytic therapy), since higher-than-normal blood pressure may be needed to maintain perfusion to the brain. Exceptions include concomitant aortic dissection, acute MI, severe heart failure, or hypertensive encephalopathy. Aggressive blood pressure lowering increases the risk of further cerebral ischemia and neurologic deterioration, as autoregulation is impaired in the ischemic bed during the acute phase of stroke. Blood pressure usually declines spontaneously as pain, agitation, and increased intracranial pressure are controlled. When drug therapy is required, useful agents include sodium nitroprusside, labetalol, and calcium antagonists (sublingual nifedipine should be avoided). Guidelines for managing hypertension during thrombolytic therapy are described on p. 29.
Myocardial infarction (MI)	MI occurs in up to 20% of patients with acute stroke and is a common cause of death between 1-4 weeks. High catecholamine levels, which accompany most strokes, may precipitate angina and MI. All patients should be carefully monitored for signs of myocardial ischemia/infarction. ECG changes following brain hemorrhage (esp. subarachnoid hemorrhage) can mimic acute myocardial ischemia/infarction, including ST-segment elevation or depression, giant upright or inverted T waves, prominent U waves, and prolonged QT interval. Cardiac markers (CK-MB, cardiac troponins) should be obtained in these cases to rule out acute MI.

Table 5.1. Treatment of Stroke-Related Complications

Complication	Comments
Arrhythmias	Sinus tachycardia, sinus bradycardia, and tachy-brady syndrome are not uncommon after stroke. Ventricular tachycardia has been reported, most often in association with a long QT interval (torsade de pointes). Cardioversion, antiarrhythmics, and pacemaker implantation are usually reserved for hemodynamic instability or symptoms.
Sepsis	Most episodes are caused by urinary tract infections (indwelling catheter, urinary retention) or pneumonia (aspiration, atelectasis). Preventive measures include intermittent bladder catheterization (preferred over continuous drainage), physical therapy with feeding guidance (feeding tube may be necessary), coughing and deep breathing exercises. A high index of suspicion for sepsis is essential, as fever, leukocytosis, and fluctuating mental status often accompany stroke without infection. Prompt antimicrobial therapy is imperative.
Upper GI bleed	Most episodes are caused by stress-related gastric mucosal damage (Cushing's ulcers). Lesions can develop rapidly and may perforate or result in severe GI bleeding. Prevention is key: gastric pH > 3.5 should be maintained with with H_2 blockers, proton pump inhibitors, or sucralfate.
Hyponatremia	Hyponatremia is an adverse prognostic factor following stroke and may be due to the syndrome of inappropriate antidiuretic hormone release (SiADH). It is important to ensure euvolemia and exclude renal, adrenal, and thyroid disorders associated with hyponatremia.
Respiratory depression, depressed consciousness	More common in hemorrhagic strokes and large strokes complicated by increased intracranial pressure. Endotracheal intubation may be needed to protect the airway, along with ventilatory support, supplemental oxygen, and bronchopulmonary toilet.
Fever	Fever is uncommon in the early hours of stroke and is associated with an adverse prognosis. Search for other causes (e.g., aspiration pneumonia, endocarditis) and treat. Administer antipyretic.
Malnutrition	Give supplemental multivitamins and thiamine. Nasogastric tube supplements are recommended if intake is still poor by day 4. A gastric feeding tube may be required.

Table 5.1. Treatment of Stroke-Related Complications

Complication	Comments
Contractures	Preventive therapy with early physical therapy is essential.
Decubitus ulcers	Meticulous attention to skin care is mandatory. Keep skin clean and dry, turn the patient frequently, and use padded boots and mattress. Wound debridement and skin grafting may be required in severe cases.

Chapter 6

Miscellaneous Topics in Cerebrovascular Disease

A. Asymptomatic Carotid Artery Stenosis

    1. Stenosis > 60%. The Asymptomatic Carotid Artery Stenosis trial (JAMA 1995;273:18) evaluated the role of endarterectomy for healthy persons with > 60% carotid artery stenosis by ultrasound. Event-free survival was improved by endarterectomy (stroke or death at 5 years: 11% with aspirin vs. 5.1% for surgery). However, surgeons were preselected, and overall surgical morbidity/mortality in the study were very low (< 3%). Also, no benefit was seen in women. For patients undergoing coronary artery bypass surgery (CABG), CABG can be performed without carotid surgery if the patient is asymptomatic or symptoms are remote. For patients with recurrent TIAs or a prior non-disabling stroke, endarterectomy should be performed either prior to or simultaneously with CABG.

    2. Stenosis < 60%. These patients should be managed with platelet inhibitors and control of risk factors for atherothrombosis (e.g., hypertension, dyslipidemia, diabetes, tobacco use, physical inactivity, obesity) (Chapters 8-13).

B. Unruptured Aneurysm. On average, rupture rates are 2-4% per year for asymptomatic aneurysms and 15% per year for symptomatic aneurysms. The risk of rupture increases with increasing size of aneurysm, and aneurysms in the posterior circulation are more likely to rupture than aneurysms in the anterior circulation (Lancet 2003;362:103-110).

Clipping, coiling, or ligation is indicated for aneurysms > 5-7 mm in diameter and for aneurysms causing progressive neurological symptoms secondary to compression. Operative mortality is low (< 2%).

C. **Carotid Endarterectomy (CEA).** CEA is strongly indicated for severe symptomatic carotid artery stenosis (> 70% narrowing) in men and women (see NASCET I, p. 122). It is also indicated for moderate symptomatic carotid artery stenosis (50-69%) in men (see NASCET II, p. 123), although the benefit is not as large. CEA is indicated for asymptomatic carotid artery stenosis (> 60%) in men if operative morbidity and mortality is less than 3%. There is no proven surgical benefit for women with symptomatic carotid artery stenosis 50-69% or asymptomatic carotid artery stenosis > 60%. Complications include death (1%), reocclusion (5-10%), and post-operative stroke (2-3%); complication rates are higher in patients with prior CEA and in diabetics. Post-operative myocardial infarction occurs in 1% of patients without coronary artery disease, in 7% of patients with stable angina, and in 17% of patients with unstable angina.

D. **Extracranial-Intracranial Bypass.** EC-IC bypass is indicated for select patients with posterior circulation occlusive disease, acute intracranial occlusions, or chronic occlusive disease with persistent ischemia shown by PET or SPECT. Superficial temporal-to-middle cerebral artery shunts are not helpful if > 6 weeks have elapsed since the ischemic insult.

E. **Carotid and Vertebral Artery Stenting.** Carotid stenting appears to be a feasible alternative to endarterectomy for carotid artery occlusive disease. Small studies indicate acceptable procedural success and complication rates, including restenosis rates < 10%. Recent results from the ARCHER and SAPPHIRE trials indicate that carotid stenting with distal embolic protection is a safe and effective alternative to carotid endarterectomy for patients at high surgical risk (Table 14.6). If confirmed in larger series, this procedure will be applicable to many patients with conditions that preclude standard operative therapy and may supplant operative therapy in some individuals. Angioplasty and stenting can also be performed successfully on stenotic vertebral arteries.

Chapter 7

Stroke Pitfalls

Pitfall: Basing treatment of stroke on brain imaging alone without a vascular work-up

Definitive treatment of stroke should be based on the vascular workup, not the CT scan or MRI alone. For example, a left frontal stroke caused by a tight carotid stenosis should be treated with revascularization, while the same stroke caused by atrial fibrillation should be treated with warfarin.

Pitfall: Basing work-up and treatment on temporal course of stroke

Work-up and treatment of stroke should focus on the vascular lesion, not the temporal course of neurological symptoms. In fact, the vascular etiology of TIA, reversible ischemic neurological deficit (RIND), stroke in evolution, and completed stroke is often the same. Furthermore, many patients with transient symptoms have small infarcts on imaging.

Pitfall: Missing a mimic of stroke or TIA

Transient neurologic deficits can be caused by structural lesions (tumor, subdural hematoma, brain abscess), metabolic disturbances (especially hypoglycemia), partial seizures, meningitis/encephalitis, psychiatric syndromes, and migraine. Stroke mimics should be considered in all patients who present with an acute neurological deficit prior to institution of treatment.

Pitfall: Missing early infarct signs on CT

Sulcal effacement, loss of the "insular ribbon," early hypodensity, and loss of gray-white differentiation (especially if large) increase the risk of hemorrhage during thrombolytic therapy. Careful assessment of the CT scan is necessary to ensure thrombolytic therapy is given to only those patients in whom potential neurological recovery outweighs the risk of intracerebral hemorrhage.

Pitfall: Underestimating the time of symptom onset for patients who wake up with a stroke

Since most strokes are painless, patients may develop strokes in their sleep and wake up with a deficit. In these cases, time of onset is unclear. Given the risks of late thrombolysis, onset time should be assumed to be the time when the patient was last observed to be well (i.e., when they went to sleep). These patients are almost always ineligible for thrombolytic therapy. In these cases diffusion-weighted MRI and MRA may help define the benefit/risk of thrombolytic therapy.

Pitfall: Overtreatment of hypertension in acute stroke

Because acutely ischemic brain tissue is unable to autoregulate, overaggressive lowering of blood pressure may lead to infarct extension and worse outcome. Hypertension should not be treated in the acute stages of stroke unless blood pressure exceeds 200/120 mmHg (or > 180/105 mmHg if thrombolytics are used).

Pitfall: Overuse of carotid endarterectomy in asymptomatic patients

Carotid endarterectomy is of proven value for symptomatic carotid disease. For patients who have > 60% carotid stenosis without symptoms, the benefits are much smaller (i.e., 1% annual reduction in subsequent risk of stroke). In asymptomatic patients, endarterectomy is indicated only if surgical risks are low (< 3%). Endarterectomy for asymptomatic women has not been shown to be beneficial.

Pitfall: Not investigating both extracranial and intracranial circulations

Embolic and thrombotic strokes can be caused by vascular lesions throughout the carotid and vertebrobasilar systems. Duplex imaging of the carotids, the most commonly ordered noninvasive test of the cerebral circulation, does not investigate the intracranial circulation. Transcranial Doppler or MRA can noninvasively detect intracranial lesions, which are more common in Asians and African-Americans.

Pitfall: Failure to distinguish severe carotid stenosis from total occlusion

Neither carotid Duplex imaging nor MRA can fully distinguish between severe stenosis (which is surgically amenable, possibly urgently) and total occlusion (where medical therapy is almost always indicated. Conventional angiography remains the test of choice.

Pitfall: Inadequate cardiac monitoring/evaluation

Silent myocardial infarction (MI) and arrhythmias are common stroke complications. MI occurs in up to 20% of patients with acute stroke and is a common cause of death at 1-4 weeks. All patients with acute stroke should undergo cardiac evaluation.

Pitfall: Not obtaining spinal fluid for patients with suspected subarachnoid hemorrhage

CT scan has 90% sensitivity for subarachnoid blood on the day of onset. Small hemorrhages can be missed, however, and CT sensitivity declines with increasing time from onset. If the CT is negative and the index of suspicion for subarachnoid hemorrhage is high, lumbar puncture is warranted.

Pitfall: Not educating patients about symptoms of stroke

More than 90% of patients with acute ischemic stroke are ineligible for lytic therapy, in large measure due to late presentation from lack of awareness of common stroke symptoms. Furthermore, many patients with diabetes, hypertension, or dyslipidemia are unaware of the silent nature of their disease or that they are at increased risk for stroke, contributing to noncompliance with medical therapy and progression of atherosclerosis. It is imperative to educate all individuals as to the warning signs of stroke, the need to seek immediate medical attention should symptoms develop, and the need to comply with primary and secondary prevention measures.

Pitfall: Not considering causes other than embolism in patients with atrial fibrillation who develop ischemic stroke

More than 25% of ischemic strokes in patients with atrial fibrillation are due to causes other than cardiogenic embolism, including intrinsic cerebrovascular disease and embolization of aortic arch atheroma. In such cases, additional measures may be required to prevent stroke recurrence (e.g., carotid revascularization).

Pitfall: Not treating patients with large artery ischemic stroke indefinitely with antiplatelet therapy

Long-term antiplatelet therapy reduces the risk of myocardial infarction and stroke by 20% in patients with previous ischemic stroke due to large artery atherothrombosis. Despite these convincing data, many eligible patients do not receive antiplatelet therapy. All patients with ischemic stroke due to large artery atherothrombosis should be treated indefinitely with either aspirin (81-325 mg once daily), clopidogrel (75 mg once daily), or combination low-dose aspirin 25 mg plus extended-release dipyridamole 200 mg twice daily. Combination aspirin plus clopidogrel can also be considered in high-risk patients, especially those at increased risk of coronary artery disease.

Pitfall: Failure to institute measures to prevent early stroke-related complications
In addition to acute MI and arrhythmias, patients with stroke are at high-risk for serious medical complications caused by prolonged bed rest and immobility (decubitus ulcer, DVT, pulmonary embolism, depression, malnutrition) and as a direct consequence of the stroke itself (increased intracranial pressure, seizures, stress-induced GI ulcers, urinary voiding problems, aspiration pneumonia). It is important to routinely institute prophylactic measures to reduce these risks, including early ambulation, bedside physical therapy, support hose or inflated stockings, subcutaneous heparin during prolonged immobilization (if not receiving IV heparin), intermittent bladder catheterization, coughing and deep breathing exercises, maintenance of gastric pH >3.5 with H_2 blockers or other drugs, meticulous attention to skin care, NG tube supplements as required, and other measures as described on pp. 40-44.

Pitfall: Failure to maintain blood pressure < 180/105 mmHg during thrombolytic therapy
To minimize the risk of intracerebral hemorrhage during/after tPA, it is imperative to maintain systolic BP < 180 mmHg and diastolic BP < 105 mmHg. IV labetalol is the antihypertensive drug of choice for this purpose (p. 29), but is not recommended in patients with significant asthma, decompensated heart failure, or high-grade conduction disturbances. Nitroprusside is generally reserved for labetalol nonresponders and those with extreme elevations in blood pressure (diastolic BP > 140 mmHg).

Pitfall: Failure to recognize lacunar stroke
Lacunar stroke presents as one of several well-defined syndromes and is

managed with long-term control of blood pressure and possibly empiric antiplatelet therapy. Anticoagulation is not indicated. Lacunar syndromes include pure motor hemiparesis, pure sensory stroke, dysarthria-clumsy-hand syndrome, ataxic hemiparesis, and isolated motor/sensory stroke (p. 24).

Pitfall: Inadequate use and dosing of HMG Co-A reductase inhibitors (statins) in patients with cerebrovascular disease
Statins reduce the risk of myocardial infarction and stroke by 20-35% in patients with atherothrombotic vascular disease and elevated LDL cholesterol levels. All patients with established cerebrovascular disease should have a lipid panel checked every 4-6 months, and a statin should be prescribed to bring LDL levels below 100 mg/dL (Chapter 12). Statins may also be useful in patients with arterial plaque/stenosis and "normal" cholesterol levels.

Pitfall: Failure to lower chronic hypertension to established targets
Proper control of hypertension reduces the risk of death from stroke, coronary artery disease, and heart failure by 15-50%. Despite these beneficial effects, only about 25% of patients with hypertension meet established guidelines. In one study, drug therapy was adjusted in only 7% of patients with blood pressure > 160/90 mmHg despite 6 or more hypertension-related visits per year (N Engl J Med 1998;339:1957). All patients should have their blood pressure lowered to at least 140/90 mmHg; lower targets have been established for patients with diabetes or chronic renal disease ($\leq$ 130/80 mmHg) (Chapter 11).

Pitfall: Not discussing smoking cessation regularly with patients
Continued cigarette smoking is a major risk factor for recurrent events in patients with cerebrovascular disease, yet less than one-third of patients discontinue smoking following a stroke. Regular and systematic discussion of the importance of smoking cessation can increase this discontinuation rate to almost 60%. Measures to assist patients willing to quit smoking and other therapeutic lifestyle changes (diet, physical activity, weight control) are described in Chapter 9.

Section 2

CEREBROVASCULAR & CARDIOVASCULAR RISK REDUCTION

Chapter 8

Overview of Cerebrovascular and Cardiovascular Risk Reduction

Atherothrombotic vascular disease is the leading cause of morbidity and mortality in developed countries, accounting for more than one-third of all deaths each year. At any one time, 12 million Americans have coronary heart disease (CHD), 4.7 million have had strokes, and millions more have claudication from peripheral arterial disease. Of the 730,000 Americans who have a stroke each year, 5-15% will have a recurrence by one year. By 5 years, up to 40% will have had a recurrent stroke and almost 50% will have died, usually from cardiovascular disease (Table 8.1). Hypertension is a major modifiable risk factor for atherosclerosis and frequently coexists with other important risk factors, including dyslipidemia, diabetes mellitus, tobacco use, obesity, and sedentary lifestyle (Table 8.2). Lifestyle modifications, pharmacologic measures, and surgical therapy can reduce the risk of stroke by 20-50%. Therapeutic lifestyle changes are recommended for all patients, while use of antiplatelet agents, anticoagulants, and arterial revascularization (endarterectomy or stents) requires individualization. Chapters 8-13 detail proven risk reduction measures aimed at halting the progression of atherosclerosis, stabilizing rupture-prone plaques, preventing arterial thromboembolism, and improving prognosis.

Table 8.1. Annual Risk of Stroke or Vascular Death for Individuals with Cerebrovascular Disease

Characteristic	Annual Risk (%)	
	Stroke	Vascular Death
General elderly male population	0.6	–
Asymptomatic carotid stenosis	1.3	3.4
Transient monocular blindness	2.2	3.5
Transient ischemic attack	3.7	2.3
Minor stroke	6.1	3.2
Major stroke	9.0	3.5
Symptomatic carotid stenosis > 70%	15.0	2.0

From: Arch Neurol 1992;49:857

Table 8.2. Modifiable Risk Factors for Ischemic Stroke

Factor	Prevalence (%)	Relative Risk of Stroke
Hypertension	25-40	3-5
Elevated total cholesterol (> 240 mg/dL)	25-40	1.8-2.6
Smoking	25	1.5
Physical inactivity	25	2.7
Obesity	18	1.8-2.4
Asymptomatic carotid stenosis > 50%	2-8	2
Alcohol > 5 drinks/day	2-5	1.6
Atrial fibrillation	1	5 (nonvalvular) 17 (valvular)

From: JAMA 2002;288:1388-1395.

Chapter 9

Therapeutic Lifestyle Changes

Diet modification, weight control, and increased physical activity are important therapeutic lifestyle changes for all patients at risk of atherothrombosis. For patients who require drug therapy for hypertension or dyslipidemia, the drug should be added to, not substituted for, diet modification and other lifestyle changes.

Diet Modification

A diet high in citrus fruits and cruciferous and green leafy vegetables was shown to protect against ischemic stroke in the Framingham study (JAMA 1995;273:1113) and the Nurses Health Study (JAMA 1999;282:1233); each increment of one daily serving reduced the risk of ischemic stroke by 6%. A diet low in saturated and trans fats and possibly high in omega-3 fats is also recommended. Light-to-moderate alcohol consumption (1 drink per week to 1 drink per day) may reduce the risk of ischemic stroke in men by 20% over 12 years (N Engl J Med 1999;341:1557), but heavy alcohol consumption (> 5 drinks/day) increases the risk of stroke. By limiting total fat, saturated fat, and dietary cholesterol in patients consuming a typical Western diet, initiation of the Therapeutic Lifestyle Changes (TLC) diet (Tables 9.1, 9.2), advocated by the National Cholesterol Education Program Adult Treatment Panel III (NCEP-ATP III) (Circulation 2002;106:3145-3421), can lower LDL cholesterol levels by 10-20%. A registered dietitian can be helpful in improving compliance. Other dietary measures to lower LDL cholesterol and reduce risk of atherothrombotic vascular disease are described in Table 9.3.

Table 9.1. Therapeutic Lifestyle Changes (TLC) Diet

Food Composition	Recommendation
Total fat	25-35% of total calories
Saturated fat*	< 7% of total calories
Polyunsaturated fat	Up to 10% of total calories
Monounsaturated fat	Up to 20% of total calories
Carbohydrates	50-60% of total calories+
Fiber	20-30 gm/d
Protein	~ 15% of total calories
Cholesterol	< 200 mg/d
Total calories	Sufficient to achieve/maintain desirable body weight

* Trans fats also raise LDL cholesterol and should be kept to a minimum
+ More than half as complex carbohydrates from whole grains, fruits, vegetables

Table 9.2. Components of the TLC Diet: Recommendations from NCEP-ATP III

Component	Evidence Statement*	Recommendations
Total fat	Unsaturated fats do not raise LDL cholesterol when substituted for carbohydrates in the diet (A2, B2).	It is not necessary to restrict total fat intake for the purpose of reducing LDL cholesterol, provided saturated fats are reduced to goal levels.
Saturated fats	High intakes of saturated fats raise LDL cholesterol and are associated with high population rates of CHD (C2). Reduction in intake of saturated fats reduces CHD risk (A1, B1).	A therapeutic diet to maximize LDL-lowering should contain < 7% of total calories as saturated fats.

* *Type of Evidence:* A: Major randomized controlled trials (RCTs); B: Smaller RCTs and meta-analyses of other clinical trials; C: Observational and metabolic studies; D: Clinical experience. *Strength of Evidence:* 1: Very strong; 2: Moderately strong; 3: Strong trend. *From:* National Cholesterol Education Program Adult Treatment Panel III Report. Circulation 2002;106:3145-3421.

Table 9.2. Components of the TLC Diet: Recommendations from NCEP-ATP III

Component	Evidence Statement*	Recommendations
Trans fats	Trans fats raise LDL cholesterol (A2). Prospective studies support an association between higher intakes of trans fatty acids and CHD incidence (C2).	Intakes of trans fats should be kept low. Liquid vegetable oil, soft margarine, and trans fat-free margarine are encouraged instead of butter, stick margarine, and shortening.
Polyunsaturated fats	Linoleic acid, a polyunsaturated fat, reduces LDL cholesterol levels when substituted for saturated fats (A1, B1). Clinical trials indicate that substitution of polyunsaturated fats for saturated fats reduces risk for CHD (A2, B2).	Polyunsaturated fats can replace saturated fat. Most polyunsaturated fats should be derived from liquid vegetable oils, semi-liquid margarines, and margarines low in trans fats. Intake can range up to 10% of total calories.
Mono-unsaturated fats	Monounsaturated fats lower LDL cholesterol relative to saturated fatty acids (A2, B2) but do not lower HDL cholesterol or raise triglycerides (A2, B2). Diets rich in monounsaturated fats provided by plant sources and rich in fruits, vegetables, and whole grains and low in saturated fats decrease CHD risk (C1).	Monounsaturated fats are one form of unsaturated fatty acid that can replace saturated fats. Intake can range up to 20% of total calories. Most monounsaturated fats should be derived from vegetable sources, including plant oils and nuts.

* *Type of Evidence:* A: Major randomized controlled trials (RCTs); B: Smaller RCTs and meta-analyses of other clinical trials; C: Observational and metabolic studies; D: Clinical experience. *Strength of Evidence:* 1: Very strong; 2: Moderately strong; 3: Strong trend. *From:* National Cholesterol Education Program Adult Treatment Panel III Report. Circulation 2002;106:3145-3421.

Table 9.2. Components of the TLC Diet: Recommendations from NCEP-ATP III

Component	Evidence Statement*	Recommendations
Cholesterol	High intakes raise LDL cholesterol (A2, B1) and the risk for CHD. Reducing intakes from high to low decreases LDL cholesterol (A2, B1).	Less than 200 mg per day of cholesterol should be consumed in the TLC Diet to maximize LDL cholesterol lowering.
Carbohydrates	When carbohydrate is substituted for saturated fats, LDL cholesterol levels fall (A2, B2). However, very high intakes of carbohydrate (>60 percent of total calories) are accompanied by a reduction in HDL cholesterol and a rise in triglyceride (B1, C1).	Daily intake should be limited to 60% of total calories in persons with the metabolic syndrome. Lower intakes (e.g., 50% of calories) should be considered for persons who have elevated triglycerides or low HDL cholesterol. Most carbohydrates should come from grain products (esp. whole grains), vegetables, fruits, fat-free/low-fat dairy.
Protein	Dietary protein in general has little effect on LDL cholesterol or other lipoprotein fractions. However, substituting soy protein for animal protein has been reported to lower LDL cholesterol.	Protein intake should constitute ~ 15% of total calories. Plant sources include legumes, dry beans, nuts, and to a lesser extent, grain products and vegetables, which are low in saturated fats/cholesterol. Animal sources of protein lower in saturated fat/cholesterol include fat-free/low-fat dairy, egg whites, fish, skinless poultry, lean meats.

* *Type of Evidence:* A: Major randomized controlled trials (RCTs); B: Smaller RCTs and meta-analyses of other clinical trials; C: Observational and metabolic studies; D: Clinical experience. *Strength of Evidence:* 1: Very strong; 2: Moderately strong; 3: Strong trend. *From:* National Cholesterol Education Program Adult Treatment Panel III Report. Circulation 2002;106:3145-3421.

**Table 9.3. Dietary Options for LDL-Lowering and Cardiovascular
Risk Reduction: Recommendations from NCEP-ATP III**

Measure	Evidence Statement*	Comments
Increasing viscous fiber in the diet	5-10 gm/d of viscous fiber reduces LDL cholesterol levels by ~ 5% (A2, B1).	The use of dietary sources of viscous fiber is a therapeutic option to enhance LDL-lowering.
Plant stanols/sterols	Intakes of 2-3 gm/d of plant stanol/sterol esters reduce LDL cholesterol by 6-15% (A2, B1).	Plant stanol/sterol esters are a therapeutic option to enhance LDL-lowering.
Soy protein	High intakes of soy protein can cause small reductions in LDL cholesterol levels, especially when it replaces animal food products (A2, B2).	Food sources containing soy protein are acceptable as replacements for animal food products containing animal fats.
n-3 (omega-3) polyunsaturated fatty acids	Higher intakes of n-3 fatty acids may reduce risk for coronary events/mortality (A2, C2).	Higher dietary intakes of n-3 fatty acids in the form of fatty fish or vegetable oils are an option for reducing CHD risk.
Folic acid and vitamins B_6 and B_{12}	There are no randomized trials to show whether lowering homocysteine levels through dietary intake or vitamins will reduce CHD risk.	ATP III endorses the Institute of Medicine RDA for dietary folate (400 mcg/d).
Antioxidants	Clinical trials have failed to show antioxidant supplements reduce CHD risk (A2).	The Institute of Medicine's RDAs for dietary antioxidants are recommended (vitamin C: 75 mg and 90 mg/d for women and men; vitamin E: 15 mg/d).

* ***Type of Evidence:*** A: Major randomized controlled trials (RCTs); B: Smaller RCTs
and meta-analyses of other clinical trials; C: Observational and metabolic studies; D:
Clinical experience. ***Strength of Evidence:*** 1: Very strong; 2: Moderately strong; 3:
Strong trend. *From:* National Cholesterol Education Program Adult Treatment Panel III
Report. Circulation 2002;106:3145-3421.

Table 9.3. Dietary Options for LDL-Lowering and Cardiovascular Risk Reduction: Recommendations from NCEP-ATP III

Measure	Evidence Statement*	Comments
Moderate alcohol intake	Moderate alcohol intake in middle-aged/older adults may reduce CHD risk (C2). High intakes of alcohol produce multiple adverse effects (C1).	Alcohol should be limited to 2 drinks per day for men and 1 drink per day for women. A drink is defined as 5 oz. wine, 12 oz. beer, or 1.5 oz. 80-proof whiskey.
Dietary sodium, potassium, and calcium	Lower salt intake lowers blood pressure or prevents its rise.	ATP III supports JNC VI recommendation of a sodium intake < 2.4 gm/d sodium or 6.4 gm/d sodium chloride and adequate intakes of dietary potassium (~ 90 mmol/day), calcium, and magnesium.
Herbal or botanical dietary supplements	Trial data are not available to support the use of herbal and botanical supplements in the prevention or treatment of heart disease.	ATP III does not recommend use of herbal or botanical dietary supplements to reduce CHD risk. Patients should be asked whether such products are being used because of potential drug interactions.
High protein, high total fat and saturated fat weight loss regimens	These diets have not been shown in controlled trials to produce long-term weight reduction, and their nutrient composition does not appear to be conducive to long-term health.	These regimens are not recommended for weight reduction in clinical practice.

* *Type of Evidence:* A: Major randomized controlled trials (RCTs); B: Smaller RCTs and meta-analyses of other clinical trials; C: Observational and metabolic studies; D: Clinical experience. *Strength of Evidence:* 1: Very strong; 2: Moderately strong; 3: Strong trend. *From:* National Cholesterol Education Program Adult Treatment Panel III Report. Circulation 2002;106:3145-3421.

Mediterranean-Style Diet

A. **Lyon Heart Study**. Increasing evidence suggests that a Mediterranean-style diet emphasizing consumption of monounsaturated and omega-3 fatty acids can play an important role in the prevention of atherothrombotic vascular disease. The Lyon Heart Study randomized 605 post-MI patients to a Mediterranean diet providing increased levels of alpha-linolenic acid (from olive oil and canola oil) or usual dietary instruction. Patients in the Mediterranean diet group were instructed to consume more fish, bread, and root and green vegetables; eat less meat; have fruit at least once daily; and use canola-based margarine and olive oil as a fat source. After 27 months, patients on the Mediterranean diet showed a 70% reduction in all-cause mortality (p = 0.03). The rate of cardiovascular death and nonfatal MI was 1.32 per 100 patient years in the treated group compared to 5.55 per 100 patient years in the control group (p = 0.001) (Lancet 1994;343:1454-9). Benefits were maintained at 4 years (Circulation 1999;99:779-85).

B. **Other Studies.** Further evidence for the vascular protective effects of omega-3 fatty acids (eicosapentaenoic acid [EPA] and docosahexaenoic acid [DHA]) from fish or fish oil supplements come from the GISSI Prevention study and Diet and Reinfarction Trial (DART). The GISSI Prevention study randomized 11,324 Italian men and women (who presumably were eating a Mediterranean diet) with MI within the preceding 3 months to omega-3 fatty acids (850-882 mg/d), vitamin E (300 mg/d), both, or neither. After 3.5 years, the omega-3 group had a significant 20% reduction in all-cause mortality and 45% reduction in sudden cardiac death (Lancet 1999;354:447-55). In DART, 2033 men with prior MI were randomized to receive different types of dietary advice to prevent another MI. After 2 years, the group told to increase their omega-3 intake by eating oily fish (e.g., salmon, herring, mackerel) at least twice weekly had a 29% reduction in overall mortality (p < 0.05) (Lancet 1989;2:757-61). Recent results from the Nurses' Health Study, which examined the risk of CHD in 84,688 previously healthy women, found that higher consumption of fish and omega-3 fatty acids reduced the risk of cardiac death by up to 45% at 16 years (JAMA

2002;287:1815-1821). Furthermore, there was an inverse relationship between fish and omega-3 fatty acid intake and thrombotic stroke: Compared to women who ate fish < 1 time per month, relative risk reductions for women who ate fish 1-3 times per month, 1 time per week, 2-4 times per week, and ≥ 5 times per week were 0.93, 0.78, 0.73, and 0.48, respectively (JAMA 2001;285:304-312). Fish consumption 1-3 times per week also reduced ischemic stroke in men (JAMA 2002;288:3130-6), and fish oil supplements have been shown to incorporate into atherosclerotic plaque and induce changes that enhance plaque stability (Lancet 2003;361:477-85). These studies suggest that the type of fat, not only the amount, affect vascular health.

C. Recommendations. Diet modification should be recommended as part of a comprehensive program to reduce vascular risk. Suggested diets are the TLC diet or a Mediterranean-style diet (Tables 9.4, 9.5).

Table 9.4. Basic Components of a Mediterranean Diet

Component	Benefits
Omega-3–rich[1] fish 1-2 times per week or omega-3 supplements[2]	Reduces all-cause mortality and sudden cardiac death post-MI; lowers triglycerides (high doses) and blood pressure; improves insulin resistance; boosts the immune system; may help prevent cancer, arthritis, depression, Alzheimer's disease.
Monounsaturated cooking oils (olive, flaxseed, or canola)	Does not increase LDL cholesterol or decrease HDL cholesterol (unlike high saturated fat or high intake of refined carbohydrate). "Metabolically neutral" calorie source for people with insulin resistance.
Fresh fruit and vegetables (5-10 servings per day); use wide variety	High concentrations of vitamins, minerals, fiber, and phytochemicals[3] help prevent heart disease, stroke, and many types of cancer (colon, stomach, prostate).
Vegetable protein from nuts and beans 1-2 times per week	Lowers LDL cholesterol; improves digestion; may reduce CHD and certain cancers. Nuts are an excellent source of protein, monounsaturated fat, fiber, and minerals. Beans contain high-quality protein, fiber, potassium, and folic acid.[4]

Table 9.4. Basic Components of a Mediterranean Diet

Component	Benefits
Limit saturated fats to < 10-20 grams per day	Saturated fats increase LDL cholesterol, which promotes atherosclerosis and increases the risk of CHD and stroke. Saturated fats are also linked to certain cancers.
Avoid trans fats	Trans fats are manufactured from vegetable oils and are used to enhance the taste and extend the shelf-life of fast foods, French fries, packaged snacks, commercial baked goods, and most margarines. Trans fats may be more atherogenic than saturated fats. Food manufacturers are not required to list trans fats on food labels; instruct patients to avoid foods with "hydrogenated" or "partially hydrogenated" vegetable oil as first or second ingredient—these contain trans fats.
Increase dietary to fiber to 20-30 grams per day	Lowers LDL cholesterol; improves insulin resistance; reduces the risk of heart disease and diabetes; protects against colon cancer, and possibly breast cancer, irritable bowel syndrome, diverticulitis and hemorrhoids; prevents constipation.
At least one source of high-quality protein with every meal	Produces satiety that lasts longer than high carbohydrate meals (reduces hunger and cravings); maintains muscle mass and bone strength. Lack of protein increases the risk of breast cancer, diabetes, and osteoporosis.

Adapted from *The Omega Diet*, by A. Simopoulos, MD

1. The typical American diet consists of an unhealthy ratio (> 15:1) of omega-6:omega-3 essential fatty acids, favoring excessive production of proinflammatory, prothrombotic, and vasoconstrictive mediators of the arachidonic acid cascade (e.g., leukotrienes, thromboxane). Increasing consumption of omega-3 essential fatty acids helps regulate inflammation, thrombogenicity, arrhythmogenicity, and vascular tone.

2. Omega-3 supplements may be considered for patients with documented CHD, especially if risk factors for sudden death are present (LV dysfunction, LVH, ventricular dysrhythmias).

3. Phytochemicals are naturally occurring chemicals found in plants—many of them plant pigments—that act as free radical scavengers and protease inhibitors, among others. Examples include lycopene, beta-carotene, indoles, thiocyanates, lutein, resveratrol, ellagic acid, genistein, and allium.

4. Folic acid lowers levels of homocysteine, a by-product of methionine metabolism associated with atherosclerosis.

Table 9.5. How to Incorporate a Mediterranean Diet into Daily Living

Step	Choose	Go Easy On	Avoid
Eat omega-3 rich food 1-2 times per week	Salmon, trout, herring, water-packed tuna, sardines, mackerel, flaxseed, spinach, purslane, fish oil supplements	Raw shellfish (due to danger of infection risk, including hepatitis A and B)	Deep-fried fish, fish sticks, fish from seriously contaminated water
Switch vegetable oils	Flaxseed oil, extra virgin cold pressed olive oil or canola oil (check the label), mayonnaise made from olive oil or canola oil	High-oleic safflower, sunflower, or soybean oil	Corn oil, safflower oil, sunflower oil, palm oil, peanut oil, other oils, mayonnaise not from olive oil/canola oil
Load up on fresh fruit and vegetables	Fresh fruit: 3-5 daily. Fresh vegetables: 4-6 daily. Use a wide variety	Fruit juice (no more than 1-2 cups per day), dried fruit, canned fruit	Vegetables or fruit prepared in heavy cream sauces or butter
Add nuts and beans 1-2 times per week	Soybeans, kidney beans, lentils, navy beans, split peas, other beans, nuts of all kinds	Heavily salted nuts	Stale or rancid nuts
Limit saturated fats to 10-20 grams per day; eat at least one source of high-quality protein with every meal	Fish, lean fresh meat with fat trimmed off, chicken and turkey without skin, nonfat or lowfat dairy products (skim milk, yogurt, low-fat cottage cheese), dark chocolate, egg whites or egg substitute, omega-3–enriched eggs	Processed lowfat meats (bologna, salami, other luncheon meats), 2% milk, "lite" cream cheese, part-skim mozzarella cheese, milk chocolate, egg yolks (3-4 per week)	Prime-grade fatty cuts of meat, goose, duck, organ meats (liver, kidneys), sausages, bacon, full-fat processed meats, hot dogs, whole milk, cream, full-fat cheeses, cream cheese, sour cream, ice cream

Table 9.5. How to Incorporate a Mediterranean Diet into Daily Living

Step	Choose	Go Easy On	Avoid
Avoid trans fats	Stanol-enriched margarine (Benecol, Take Control)	Commercial peanut butter, water crackers and other crackers that contain no fat, bagels	Fast food, French fries and other deep-fried food, chips and other packaged snacks, most commercial baked goods, most margarines
Add more fiber; aim for 20-30 grams per day	Whole-grain breads and cereals, oats, brown rice, whole grain pasta, potatoes with skin (baked, boiled, steamed), whole-grain bagels	Pasta, white rice, mashed instant potatoes, plain bagels, dinner rolls, egg noodles	Sweetened cereals, white bread, crackers, table sugar, honey, syrup, candy, highly processed foods, especially those with white flour/sugar
Drink at least 64 ounces of water per day	Drink 8 glasses of pure, non-chlorinated water per day. Additional drinks: skim milk (up to 4 glasses); pure fruit juice (up to 2 glasses); tea, especially green tea (up to 4 cups); smoothie with plain nonfat yogurt and fresh fruit	Coffee (regular or decaf), 1% or 2% milk, artificially sweetened fruit juice (the tip-off is "corn syrup" in the label), sports drinks, soft drinks, alcohol (no more than 1 drink daily for women, 2 drinks daily for men)	Sugared soft drinks, milkshakes, excess alcohol

Physical Activity

A. **Overview.** Physical inactivity increases the risk of heart disease and stroke as much as cigarette smoking, yet more than 70% of adults get little or no exercise. All patients should be encouraged to obtain 30-45 minutes of aerobic activity on most days of the week. Regular exercise that increases heart rate to 60-80% of maximal peak heart rate for 30 minutes on all or most days of the week can raise HDL cholesterol levels by up to 30% and can prevent or improve hypertension, insulin resistance and type 2 diabetes, obesity, anxiety, and depression. Regular exercise can also help smokers quit, reduce the risk of MI and stroke by 50% or more, reduce the risk of death post-MI by 25%, and improve functional capacity in patients with claudication from peripheral arterial disease. Noncardiac benefits include a lower risk of cancer (colon, prostate, breast) and salutary effects on osteoporosis, arthritis, constipation, insomnia, and postmenopausal symptoms.

B. **Amount of Exercise.** Traditionally, exercise programs have focused exclusively on aerobic activities such as walking, running, cycling, and swimming. Recent data suggest that a strength (weight) training program is an important supplement to aerobic exercise, increasing muscle mass (which increases metabolic rate), improving insulin sensitivity, and helping maintain bone and muscular strength to prevent injuries and disability. Physical activity does not need to be performed in a traditional structured exercise program to provide health benefits, and a lifestyle-based exercise program incorporating physical activity into daily living is effective at improving risk factors, weight, and long-term cardiovascular prognosis (JAMA 1999;281:327-34). This can be accomplished by encouraging patients to use the stairs, walk whenever possible, garden, play actively with children, etc. Examples of moderate physical activity from the Surgeon General's Report on Physical Activity and Health (JAMA 1996;276:522) include:
- Wash and wax a car, or wash windows or floors for 45 minutes
- Garden, dance fast (social), or rake for 30 minutes
- Walk 1¾ miles in 35 minutes (20 min/mile)
- Push a stroller 1½ miles or bicycle 5 miles in 30 minutes

- Stairwalk, shovel snow, or jump rope for 15 minutes

Exercise should not be exhausting, but it does need to be invigorating and should increase heart rate. Individuals are exercising at the right level of intensity if they can talk without gasping for breath but do not have enough breath to sing (e.g., brisk walking at a pace of 3-4 miles per hour, like walking to catch a bus). For motivated patients able and willing to take their pulse, a reasonable goal is to exercise at 60-80% of maximal heart rate (220 – age [years]). Additionally, exercise does not need to be done all at one time during the day to receive health benefits. The important factor is to accumulate at least 30 minutes of moderate physical activity all or most days of the week (which can be split in three 10-minute blocks). Health benefits may plateau at 3500 kcal per week, the equivalent of moderately intense jogging or bicycling for 1 hour per day.

C. Stress Testing. Patients with cardiovascular or respiratory disease, or sedentary patients with multiple CHD risk factors interested in participating in a vigorous exercise program should be considered for stress testing.

Weight Control

A. Overview. An estimated 65% of U.S. adults (127 million) are overweight or obese, a number that has tripled over the last 2 decades. Overweight and obesity increase the risk of all-cause mortality, and they increase morbidity from stroke, hypertension, dyslipidemia, type 2 diabetes, CHD, stroke, gallbladder disease, osteoarthritis, sleep apnea, respiratory problems, and cancer (endometrial, breast, prostate, colon). Overweight adults are also more likely to have overweight children. Weight control improves blood pressure, triglycerides, LDL and HDL cholesterol, blood glucose, and hemoglobin A_{1c} levels in type 2 diabetics. The following information summarizes key recommendations from the NHLBI Clinical Guidelines for the Identification, Evaluation, and Treatment of Overweight and Obesity in Adults (Obesity Res 1998;6:51S-209S; Executive Summary, Arch Intern Med 1998;158:1855-67).

B. **Classification of Obesity.** All patients should be stratified by body mass index (BMI) to assess overweight/obesity and by waist circumference to assess abdominal fat content, which identifies increased risk for CHD independent of BMI and is a criterion for diagnosis of the metabolic syndrome (Table 9.6).

C. **Evaluation of Obesity.** Patient medications should be reviewed to see if adjustments or substitutions can be made to drugs associated with weight gain, including antidepressants, glucocorticoids, phenothiazines, lithium, cyproheptadine, sulfonylureas, and insulin. It is also important to examine patients for features suggestive of Cushing's syndrome (truncal obesity, moon facies, ecchymosis, muscle atrophy, edema, striae, acne, hirsutism, osteoporosis, glucose intolerance, hypokalemia) or hypothyroidism (weakness, fatigue, cold intolerance, constipation, dry skin, bradycardia, hyporeflexia). Patients with suspected sleep apnea (cessation of breathing during sleep, snoring, restless sleep, excessive daytime sleepiness, headaches, memory impairment) should be referred to a specialist.

D. **Treatment of Obesity.** The treatment of overweight/obesity requires a combination of dietary restriction, increased physical activity, and behavior modification; patients requiring additional measures may benefit from drug therapy and weight loss surgery (refractory cases). Total caloric intake and energy expenditure (physical activity) should be adjusted to achieve and maintain a desirable body weight (BMI 21-25 kg/m^2) and waist circumference (< 102 cm in men, < 88 cm in women). A reasonable initial goal is to reduce body weight by 10% over 6 months, which typically requires calorie deficits of 300-500 kcal/d in patients with BMIs of 27-35 kg/m^2 (0.5-1 lb/week) and 500-1000 kcal/d (1-2 lb/week) in patients with BMIs ≥ 35 kg/m^2. Further weight loss can be considered once this goal is achieved. Calorie deficits are best accomplished through a combination of dietary restriction and increased physical activity.

Table 9.6. Classification of Overweight and Obesity

Category	BMI*	Waist Circumference†	Risk for Type 2 Diabetes, Hypertension, CHD
Underweight	< 18.5	N or ↑	N
Normal	18.5 - 24.9	N or ↑	N or ↑
Overweight	25.0 - 29.9	N ↑	Increased High
Obesity, class I	30.0 - 34.9	N ↑	High Very high
II	35.0 - 39.9	N or ↑	Very high
III	≥ 40.0	N or ↑	Extremely high

BMI = body mass index, CHD = coronary heart disease, N = not elevated

* Body mass index = weight in kilograms divided by height in meters squared (kg/m^2). Estimated BMI using nonmetric measurements = (weight in pounds x 703) divided by height in inches squared

† Increased waist circumference: men > 102 cm (> 40 inches); women > 88 cm (> 35 inches). Increased waist circumference can be a marker for increased risk even in persons of normal weight

Adapted from: NHLBI Guideline Report (Obesity Res 1998;6:51S-209S)

1. **Dietary Restriction.** Calorie deficits of 500-1000 kcal/d usually require a diet providing 1000-1200 kcal/d for women and 1200-1500 kcal/d for men. Low-carbohydrate and other "fad" diets may facilitate early weight loss, but these diets are difficult to maintain, frequently unhealthy, and often result in diminished self-esteem as weight is inevitably regained. The best approach to diet is to eat smaller portions of a well-rounded (TLC or Mediterranean-style) diet (pp. 54-65).

2. **Increased Physical Activity.** Increased physical activity is an essential component of an effective weight loss program, leading to calorie deficits and improvements in cardiovascular risk factors, mood, and self-esteem. Walking is an excellent option for obese patients, initially at 10 minutes per day 3 times weekly, and building to 30-45 minutes per day on most or all days of the week. Ordinary household tasks can

also lead to substantial calorie deficits. A stress test should be considered prior to initiating an exercise program in individuals with known cardiovascular or pulmonary disease, and for sedentary males > 40 years or females > 50 years with 2 or more cardiovascular risk factors.

3. **Behavior Therapy.** It is essential to communicate encouragement, support, and understanding in order to optimize compliance. Other useful behavior modification techniques include self-monitoring (food consumption and exercise), stress management (coping strategies, relaxation techniques, drug therapy), problem solving (coping with urges and cravings), contingency management (rewarding achieved goals), cognitive restructuring (changing unrealistic goals and improving self-image), and social support (positive reinforcement).

4. **Drug Therapy (Table 9.7).** Pharmacotherapy can be a useful adjunct to dietary restriction, increased physical activity, and behavior modification, but is unlikely to be effective without lifestyle modification. Drug therapy is especially useful for patients with BMIs $\geq$ 30 kg/m^2 or $\geq$ 27 kg/m^2 in the presence of other risk factors (hypertension, dyslipidemia, type 2 diabetes, CHD, sleep apnea).

5. **Weight Loss Surgery.** Gastrointestinal surgery (gastric restriction or bypass) should be reserved for motivated patients with extreme obesity (BMI $\geq$ 40 kg/m^2 or $\geq$ 35 kg/m^2 with comorbid conditions) despite nonsurgical intervention. Lifelong medical monitoring and nutritional supplementation with minerals and vitamins are required.

Table 9.7. Antiobesity Drugs Approved by the FDA

	Sibutramine HCL (Meridia)	Orlistat (Xenical)
Drug class	Mixed neurotransmitter reuptake inhibitor (norepinephrine, serotonin, dopamine)	Lipase inhibitor; inhibits dietary fat absorption by 30%
Indications	Adjunct to diet in the management of obesity in patients with BMI ≥ 30 kg/m^2 or ≥ 27 kg/m^2 in the presence of other risk factors	Same as sibutramine
Dose	Initial dose: 10 mg once daily. After 4 weeks, may titrate to 15 mg once daily. Not recommended for children < 16 years	One 120-mg capsule 3 times daily with each main meal containing fat, taken during or up to 1 hour after meals. If a meal is missed or has no fat, the dose can be omitted. Not recommended in children
Contra-indications	During or within 2 weeks of MAO inhibitors (e.g., phenelzine, selegiline); concomitant use of centrally acting appetite suppressants; anorexia nervosa. Not recommended in poorly controlled hypertension, CHD, heart failure, arrhythmias, or stroke	Chronic malabsorption syndrome or cholestasis
Precautions	Not recommended in severe renal impairment or hepatic dysfunction. Check blood pressure and pulse at baseline and regularly during therapy; discontinue or reduce dose for sustained increases in either. Caution if history of seizures (discontinue if occur), hypertension, narrow-angle glaucoma, elderly. Pregnancy (Cat. C); not recommended in nursing mothers	History of hyperoxaluria; calcium oxalate nephrolithiasis. Weight loss may affect doses needed for antidiabetic drugs (monitor). Pregnancy (Cat.B); not recommended in nursing mothers

Table 9.7. Antiobesity Drugs Approved by the FDA

	Sibutramine HCL (Meridia)	Orlistat (Xenical)
Drug interactions	Avoid within 2 weeks of MAO inhibitors. Caution with other CNS drugs. Do not coadminister other serotonergic drugs (e.g., sumatriptan, SSRIs, venlafaxine), dihydroergotamine, some opioids (e.g., dextromethorphan, meperidine), lithium, or tryptophan due to possible serotonin syndrome (neuroexcitatory). Do not coadminister other drugs that can raise BP or pulse. Possible interaction with ketoconazole, erythromycin, others metabolized by CYP3A4. Not recommended with excess alcohol	May decrease absorption of fat-soluble vitamins and beta-carotene; supplement diet with a multivitamin and separate dosing by at least 2 hours. Monitor warfarin (INR), cyclosporine levels
Side effects	Dry mouth, anorexia, insomnia, constipation, headache, increased appetite, dizziness, nervousness, GI upset, increased BP/pulse, mydriasis	GI effects: oily spotting, flatus with discharge, fecal urgency, fatty/oily stools, oily evacuation, increased defecation, fecal incontinence
How supplied	5 mg, 10 mg, 15 mg capsules	120 mg capsules

Smoking Cessation

A. **Overview.** Tobacco use is one of the most important risk factors for stroke
and CHD and is the most preventable cause of death in the U.S. Each year,
400,000 deaths are attributable to tobacco use, more than alcohol abuse,
automobile accidents, AIDS, homicide, suicide, heroin, and cocaine
combined. Compared to age-matched nonsmokers, persons who smoke 1
pack of cigarettes per day are 14 times more likely to die from cancer of
the lung, throat or mouth; 4 times more likely to die from cancer of the
esophagus; twice as likely to suffer an MI or stroke; and twice as likely to
die from heart disease or cancer of the bladder. At any age, the risk of
death is doubled in smokers compared with nonsmoking age-matched
controls. Despite these statistics, few physicians routinely ask patients
about cigarette smoking or offer counseling about smoking cessation. The
increased vascular risk attributable to smoking returns to baseline soon
after cessation of tobacco use, emphasizing the importance of intervention.
By 12-18 months, most of the increased risk has disappeared, and by 3-5
years, the risk of vascular events is no different than that of a nonsmoker.
As a physician, there is virtually nothing more effective at improving a
patient's long-term prognosis than convincing and helping him or her to
stop smoking. If a physician discusses this topic even briefly with the
smoker and makes a strong statement about the medical necessity of
discontinuing this habit, a person's chances of permanent cessation of
smoking is doubled. The use of bupropion hydrochloride (Zyban) and
nicotine replacement therapy (NRT) also increases the chances of
successful smoking cessation.

B. **Guidelines.** The U.S. Public Health Service issued a clinical practice
guideline for treating tobacco use and dependence (JAMA 2000;283:3244).
The report concluded that every patient should be asked about cigarette
smoking at *every* visit, and that all smokers should be strongly encouraged
to stop and offered NRT and/or bupropion hydrochloride. The following
strategies were recommended to help patients willing to quit smoking:
- **Step 1: Systematically identify all tobacco users at every visit.** Place
  tobacco-use status stickers on all patient charts.

- **Step 2: Strongly urge all tobacco users to quit.** Advice should be clear, strong, and personalized: "I think it is important for you to quit smoking now, and I can help you." "As your clinician, I need you to know that quitting smoking is the most important thing you can do to protect your health now and in the future. The clinic staff and I will help you." Tie tobacco use to the patient's current health/illness, its social and economic costs, and its impact on children and family.

- **Step 3: Determine willingness to make a quit attempt.** If the patient is willing to make a quit attempt, assist the patient in quitting or refer the patient to a quit-smoking program. If the patient is unwilling to make a quit attempt, provide a motivational intervention.

- **Step 4: Aid the patient in quitting** (Tables 9.8, 9.9).

- **Step 5: Schedule follow-up contact.** Follow-up contact should occur soon after the quit date, preferably during the first week. A second follow-up contact is recommended within the first month. Congratulate success during follow-up contact. If tobacco use has occurred, review the circumstances and elicit a recommitment to total abstinence. Remind the patient that a lapse can be used as a learning experience. Identify problems already encountered and anticipate challenges in the immediate future. Assess pharmacotherapy use and problems, and consider use or referral to more intensive treatment.

For patients who continue to smoke, it is important to recognize interactions between cardiovascular drug therapy and cigarette smoking. These include increased metabolism/elimination of anticoagulants and beta-blockers, possibly requiring higher doses, and decreased diuretic effect due to increased secretion of vasopressin.

Table 9.8. Strategies to Assist Patients Willing to Quit Smoking

Step	Strategies for Implementation
Help the patient with a quit plan	<ul><li>Set a quit date, ideally within 2 weeks.</li><li>Tell family, friends, and coworkers about quitting; request understanding and support.</li><li>Anticipate withdrawal symptoms and discuss ways to resist urges and cravings (clean the house; take a 5-minute walk; do stretching exercises; put a toothpick, cinnamon gum, or lemon drop in mouth; take several slow deep breaths; brush teeth; call a nonsmoking friend and talk).</li><li>Remove tobacco products from your environment. Throw out ashtrays. Clean clothes, car, carpets.</li><li>Learn as much about how to quit smoking as possible. Useful sources for reading materials include:<ul><li>– American Heart Association, 7272 Greenville Avenue, Dallas, TX 75231, (800) 242-8721; www.americanheart.org</li><li>– American Cancer Society, 1599 Clifton Road, NE, Atlanta, GA 30329, (800) 227-2345; www.cancer.org</li><li>– American Lung Association, 1740 Broadway, 14th floor, New York, NY 10019, (800) 586-4872; www.lungusa.org</li><li>– National Cancer Institute, Bethesda, MD 20894, (202) 4-CANCER (422-6237); www.nci.nih.gov</li><li>– *For pregnant women:* American College of Obstetricians and Gynecologists, 409 12th Street, SW, Washington, DC 20024, (202) 638-5577; www.acog.org</li></ul></li></ul>
Provide practical counseling	<ul><li>Total abstinence is essential. "Not even a single puff after the quit date."</li><li>Identify what helped and hurt in previous quit attempts.</li><li>Discuss challenges/triggers and how to overcome them.</li><li>Since alcohol can cause relapse, the patient should consider limiting/abstaining from alcohol while quitting.</li><li>Patients should encourage housemates to quit with them or not to smoke in their presence.</li><li>Provide a supportive clinical environment while encouraging the patient during the quit attempt: "My office staff and I are available to assist you."</li></ul>

Table 9.8. Strategies to Assist Patients Willing to Quit Smoking

Step	Strategies for Implementation
Recommend approved drug therapy	• Recommend the use of first-line drug therapy (Table 9.9) to all smokers trying to quit, except in special circumstances (e.g., medical contraindications, those smoking fewer than 10 cigarettes/day, pregnant/breastfeeding women, adolescent smokers). If drug therapy is used with lighter smokers (10-15 cigarettes/day), consider reducing the dose of NRT; no dosage adjustment is necessary for sustained-release bupropion hydrochloride.
	• Some studies suggest that bupropion may be more effective than NRT for achieving permanent cessation of tobacco use, and that some synergism between the two approaches may exist. There are insufficient data to rank-order these medications, so initial therapy must be guided by factors such as clinician familiarity with the medications, contraindications for selected patients, patient preference, previous patient experience with a specific therapy (positive or negative), and patient characteristics (e.g., history of depression, concerns about weight gain). Sustained-release bupropion hydrochloride and NRT, in particular nicotine gum, have been shown to delay but not prevent weight gain. Sustained-release bupropion hydrochloride and nortriptyline hydrochloride are particularly well-suited for patients with a history of depression.
	• There is evidence that combining the nicotine patch with either nicotine gum or nicotine nasal spray increases long-term abstinence rates over those produced by a single form of NRT, based on a meta-analysis.
	• The nicotine patch in particular is safe in patients with cardiovascular disease. However, the safety of these products has not been established for the immediate post-MI period or in patients with severe or unstable angina.
	• Long-term therapy may be helpful for smokers who report persistent withdrawal symptoms. A minority of individuals who successfully quit smoking use NRT medications (gum, nasal spray, inhaler) long term. The long-term use of these medications does not present a known health risk, and the FDA has approved the use of sustained-release bupropion hydrochloride for long-term maintenance.
	• Clonidine and nortriptyline may be considered when first-line medications are contraindicated or not helpful.

Adapted from: The U.S. Public Health Service Clinical Practice Guidelines for Treating Tobacco Use and Dependence (JAMA 2000;283:3244-54)

Table 9.9. Drug Therapy for Smoking Cessation*

Therapy	Precautions	Adverse Effects	Dosage and Duration
First-line *Bupropion HCl (Zyban)*	Contraindicated in patients with a history of seizures, eating disorder, MAO inhibitor within 14 days	Insomnia, dry mouth, seizures	150 mg every morning for 3 days, then 150 mg twice daily. Begin treatment 1-2 weeks prior to quit date. Treat for 7-12 weeks. Maintenance therapy may be needed for up to 6 months
Nicotine gum (Nicorette)	Concurrent cigarette smoking is contraindicated due to the risk of nicotine overdose	Mouth soreness, dyspepsia	For < 25 cigarettes/d: 2-mg gum. For ≥ 25 cigarettes/d: 4-mg gum. Weeks 1-6: 1 piece every 1-2 hours (at least 9 pieces/d); weeks 7-9: 1 piece every 2-4 hours; weeks 10-12: 1 piece every 4-8 hours
Nicotine inhaler (Nicotrol inhaler)		Irritation of mouth and throat, coughing, rhinitis	6-16 cartridges/d x 12 weeks followed by a 6- to 12-week weaning period, if needed. Best effect achieved by continuous puffing (20 minutes)
Nicotine nasal spray (Nicotrol NS)		Nasal irritation	8-40 doses/d for 3 months. Each dose consists of 2 sprays (1 per nostril) and delivers 1 mg of nicotine to the nasal mucosa
Nicotine patch (Nicoderm CQ; Nicotrol)		Local skin reaction, insomnia	*Nicoderm CQ:* 21 mg/24 h (6 weeks), then 14 mg/24 h (2 weeks), then 7 mg/24 h (2 weeks). Light smokers (≤ 10 cigarettes/d) should start with 14-mg dose. *Nicotrol patch:* 15 mg/24 h (6 weeks)
Second-line *Clonidine*	Rebound hypertension	Dry mouth, drowsiness, dizziness, sedation	0.15-0.75 mg/d for 3-10 weeks
Nortriptyline	Risk of arrhythmias	Sedation, dry mouth	75-100 mg/d for 12 weeks

* See package inserts for additional information. First-line therapies have been approved for smoking cessation by the Food and Drug Administration; second-line therapies have not. Adapted from: The U.S. Public Health Service Clinical Practice Guidelines for Treating Tobacco Use and Dependence (JAMA 2000;283:3224-54).

Chapter 10

Antiplatelet and Antithrombotic Therapy for the Prevention of Recurrent Ischemic Stroke

More than 700,000 Americans have a stroke each year. By one year, 5-15% will have had a recurrent stroke; by 5 years, 25-40% will have had a recurrent stroke and 15-25% will have died from a vascular cause. Ischemic stroke accounts for 80% of all strokes, and many ischemic strokes are caused by large artery atherothrombosis (Chapter 1). In addition to therapeutic lifestyle changes and control of dyslipidemia, hypertension, and diabetes mellitus, the risk of vascular events in patients with ischemic stroke may be reduced by pharmacologic measures aimed at reducing the risk of atherothrombosis.

Antiplatelet Therapy

A. **Atherothrombosis as a Systemic Disease.** Atherothrombosis is a generalized process, often involving multiple arterial beds (cerebral, coronary, peripheral) at the same time. Clinical trials show that 25-45% of patients with ischemic stroke have coexistent coronary artery disease, and myocardial infarction is a leading cause of death long term.

B. **Role of the Platelet in Ischemic Stroke.** Atherothrombosis is a dynamic, progressive process of arterial injury, thrombosis, and repair. The resulting atherosclerotic plaque progresses through phases leading to progressive stenosis or acute plaque rupture and intravascular thrombosis, the common underlying mechanism of ischemic stroke, unstable angina, and acute MI (Figure 10.1). Nonobstructive plaques with extensive inflammation (stimulated by oxidized lipoproteins in the vessel wall), lipid-rich cores, and thin fibrous caps are more prone to ulceration and thrombosis than long-standing obstructive lesions with extensive calcification and thick fibrous caps comprised of dense collagenous tissue. Platelet adhesion, activation, and aggregation are central to arterial thrombosis, and antiplatelet therapy has been shown to reduce ischemic stroke, nonfatal MI, or vascular death by 25% in high-risk patients (BMJ

2002;324:71-86). Aspirin is the least expensive and most widely studied antiplatelet agent. Compared to aspirin, the thienopyridines (clopidogrel, ticlopidine), which block ADP-mediated platelet activation and subsequent aggregation, reduced the risk of recurrent stroke by 14% in a meta-analysis of 4 randomized trials (Stroke 2000;31:1779-84). Dual antiplatelet therapy, utilizing two antiplatelet agents with different mechanisms of actions, may be more effective at preventing vascular events than monotherapy. All patients with previous TIA or ischemic stroke due to large artery atherothrombosis should be treated with antiplatelet therapy unless there is a specific contraindication. Antiplatelet therapy has not been shown to reduce the risk of initial stroke in persons without vascular disease or risk factors for atherosclerosis.

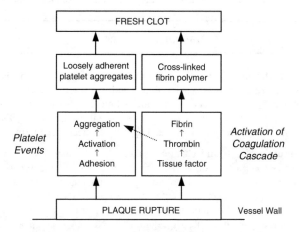

Figure 10.1. Pathophysiology of Acute Ischemic Stroke

Intravascular thrombosis is central to the pathogenesis of acute ischemic stroke. Plaque rupture exposes circulating blood to vessel wall contents, which rapidly induces clot formation via activation of two complementary systems: platelets and the coagulation cascade. The mechanism of action of antiplatelet agents is shown in Figure 10.2.

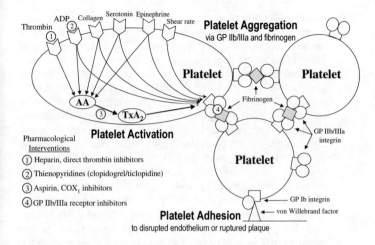

Figure 10.2. Mechanism of Antiplatelet Therapy

AA = arachadonic acid, ADP = adenosine diphosphate, COX = cyclooxygenase, GP = glycoprotein, TXA_2 = thromboxane A_2. Plaque rupture induces platelets to proceed through adhesion, activation, and aggregation. Platelet adhesion is initiated by the binding of von Willebrand factor (vWF), an adhesive glycoprotein released from the injured vessel wall, to the platelet glycoprotein (GP) Ib receptor. Platelets are exposed to multiple agonists at the same time (ADP, TXA_2, epinephrine, thrombin, serotonin, collagen), which trigger a series of events within the platelet, including increased cytosolic calcium, cell shape changes, phosphorylation of proteins, release of granules and lysosomes, arachidonic acid metabolism, and conformational change in the GP IIb/IIIa receptor complex so that it becomes expressed and active on the platelet surface. 50,000-80,000 GP IIb/IIIa receptors reside on the surface of activated platelets. Fibrinogen is the most important ligand of the GP IIb/IIIa receptor and can bind two GP IIa/IIIb receptors simultaneously, creating a molecular platelet-to-platelet bridge. Aspirin blocks the formation of thromboxane A_2 through irreversible acetylation of platelet cyclooxygenase. Clopidogrel and ticlopidine irreversibly modify the platelet ADP receptor, interfering with binding of ADP to its receptor and ADP-mediated activation of the GP IIb/IIIa receptor. Dipyridamole is a phosphodiesterase inhibitor that raises platelet levels of cyclic AMP. Adapted from: Peterson M, Dangas G, Fuster V, in: *The Manual of Interventional Cardiology, 3rd ed.,* Physicians' Press, Royal Oak, MI.

C. Antiplatelet Monotherapy

1. **Aspirin.** Aspirin exerts its antiplatelet effects by blocking the formation of thromboxane A_2 through irreversible acetylation of platelet cyclooxygenase, decreasing the likelihood that an occlusive thrombus will form at the site of an inflamed, ulcerated atherosclerotic plaque. Enzyme inhibition lasts for the lifespan of the platelet (~ 10 days). Aspirin does not prevent atherosclerosis, platelet adhesion, or platelet aggregation in response to ADP, collagen, thrombin, or epinephrine. The Antithrombotic Trialists' Collaborative (ATC) overview of randomized trials of antiplatelet therapy, comprising more than 210,000 patients in 287 studies, found that aspirin reduced the risk of vascular events in high-risk patients, including recurrent stroke, by 22% (BMJ 2002;324:71-86). The optimal dose of aspirin is not known, although ATC found that doses of 75-150 mg seem to be as effective as higher doses for long term therapy. Doses in excess of 325 mg/d are associated with increased risk of gastrointestinal bleeding in a dose-dependent fashion. Enteric-coated or buffered forms of aspirin are no less likely to cause gastrointestinal bleeding than soluble aspirin. Low-dose aspirin (75-162 mg) should be considered for patients with a history of serious bleeding, especially from the gastrointestinal tract, and aspirin should not be given for a minimum of 24 hours after thrombolytic therapy for ischemic stroke, due to an increased risk of intracranial bleeding. A significant minority of patients with coronary artery disease or prior stroke are aspirin resistant (Circulation 2000;18:II-418; Thromb Haemost 2002;88:711-5), which may increase the risk of recurrent vascular events (Circulation 2002;105:1650-5; Thromb Res 1993;71:397-403). Patients who have a recurrent TIA or ischemic stroke while on aspirin should be treated with clopidogrel or dual antiplatelet therapy.

2. **Clopidogrel.** Clopidogrel is an inhibitor of ADP-induced platelet activation and subsequent aggregation, acting by irreversible binding to the platelet $P2Y_{12}$ receptor and of the subsequent ADP-mediated activation of the platelet GP IIb/IIIa receptor complex. Clopidogrel irreversibly modifies the platelet ADP receptor, so that platelets exposed to clopidogrel are affected for the remainder of their lifespan. Compared to ticlopidine, another thienopyridine derivative,

clopidogrel has a longer duration of action, faster onset of action, and is better tolerated with fewer adverse hematologic effects (Thromb Haemost 1996;76:939-43; Platelets 1993;4:252-61). In the Clopidogrel vs. Aspirin in Patients at Risk for Ischemic Events (CAPRIE) trial, 19,185 patients with atherosclerotic vascular disease (MI within 35 days, ischemic stroke within 6 months, or established peripheral arterial disease) were randomized to clopidogrel (75 mg/d) or aspirin (325 mg/d). At a mean follow-up of 1.9 years, clopidogrel was more effective than aspirin at reducing the combined endpoint of stroke, MI, or vascular death (relative risk reduction 8.7%; p = 0.043) (Lancet 1996;348:1329). Clopidogrel resulted in slightly fewer bleeding complications, and there was no difference in the incidence of severe neutropenia between groups. In a meta-analysis of 4 randomized trials, thienopyridines (clopidogrel, ticlopidine) reduced the relative risk of recurrent stroke by 14% compared to aspirin (Stroke 2000;1779-84). Clopidogrel is approved for the reduction of atherothrombotic events (MI, ischemic stroke, vascular death) in patients with recent MI, recent stroke, or established peripheral arterial disease, and is an excellent choice for patients with cerebrovascular disease who require antiplatelet therapy. The safety profile of clopidogrel is similar to aspirin and better than ticlopidine, with a rare incidence (~ 4 per million) of thrombotic thrombocytopenic purpura (N Engl J Med 2000;342:1773-7). Combination antiplatelet therapy with aspirin plus clopidogrel has been shown to reduce vascular events in patients with ischemic heart disease compared to aspirin alone and is under investigation for patients with previous TIA or ischemic stroke (pp. 82-84).

3. **Ticlopidine.** Ticlopidine is similar to clopidogrel in structure and mechanism of action, and has been shown to reduce the risk of recurrent stroke by > 20% compared to aspirin in CATS and TASS but not in AAASPS (pp. 114-116). Efficacy is limited by adverse effects, including rash, diarrhea, neutropenia (2.3-3.4%), thrombocytopenia, and thrombotic thrombocytopenic purpura (1 in 2000-4000 patients) (Ann Intern Med 19998;128:541-4). Because of its superior safety profile, clopidogrel has replaced ticlopidine in the management of patients with atherothrombotic disease.

B. **Combination Antiplatelet Therapy.** Ex-vivo platelet aggregation studies and clinical trials indicate that utilizing two antiplatelet agents with different mechanisms of actions may be more effective at preventing platelet aggregation and vascular events than single-agent therapy.

   1. **Combination aspirin plus dipyridamole.** Among 10,404 patients in 25 trials comparing aspirin plus dipyridamole vs. aspirin alone, combination therapy resulted in a nonsignificant 6% reduction in vascular events (Antithrombotic Trialists' Collaboration: BMJ 2003;324:71-86). In the European Stroke Prevention Study (ESPS)-2, 6602 patients with ischemic stroke (76%) or TIA (24%) within 3 months were randomized to twice daily dosing of low-dose aspirin/extended-release dipyridamole (25mg/200mg), either agent alone, or placebo. At 24 months, combination therapy reduced the risk of stroke by 23.1% compared to aspirin alone (p = 0.006), by 24.7% compared to dipyridamole alone (p = 0.002), and by 37.0% compared to placebo (p < 0.001)(J Neurol Sci 1996;143:1-13). Aspirin plus dipyridamole did not, however, reduce the risk of MI or death compared to either agent alone. The most common side effect of dipyridamole is headache. The currently available preparation (aspirin 25 mg plus dipyridamole 200 mg) is given as one capsule twice daily and is approved for the prevention of recurrent stroke in patients with TIA or prior atherothrombotic ischemic stroke. The low dose of aspirin (50 mg/d) in this preparation does not provide adequate protection against recurrent MI or angina pectoris.

   2. **Combination aspirin plus clopidogrel.** This combination has recently been shown to reduce vascular events in two randomized cardiovascular trials and is under investigation in high-risk patients with recent TIA or stroke. It has also been shown to reduce ex-vivo platelet aggregation to a greater extent than aspirin alone or aspirin plus dipyridamole (presented at American Heart Association Scientific Sessions, 2002).

      a. **Treatment of acute coronary syndromes (ACS).** In the Clopidogrel in Unstable angina to prevent Recurrent Events (CURE) trial, 12,562 patients with unstable angina or non-ST-elevation MI were treated with aspirin (75-325 mg/d) and randomized to clopidogrel (300 mg loading dose followed by 75 mg/d) or placebo for up to 12 months (average 9 months). Patients receiving clopidogrel had a highly significant 20% reduction in the primary composite endpoint of cardiovascular death, MI, or stroke (9.3% vs. 11.5%, p < 0.001) (N Engl J Med 2001;345:494-502). Benefits were independent of concomitant cardiovascular medications, including ACE inhibitors and lipid-lowering therapy. Among 506 patients with prior stroke, there was a trend toward a reduction in the primary endpoint in the clopidogrel group (17.9% vs. 22.4%, RRR 26%, 95% CI 0.50-1.10). There was a 1% absolute increase in major bleeding complications with clopidogrel, but there was no increase in hemorrhagic or fatal bleeding. (Bleeding was lower in patients receiving < 100 mg/d aspirin compared to patients receiving > 300 mg/d.) In CURE, 2658 of 12,562 patients underwent percutaneous coronary intervention (PCI). Patients received study drug (clopidogrel or placebo) for a median of 10 days prior to PCI, open-label clopidogrel for 2-4 weeks after PCI, then resumption of study drug for a mean of 8 months. Clopidogrel resulted in an overall (before and after PCI) reduction in cardiovascular death or MI by 31% (8.8% vs. 12.6%, p = 0.002) (Lancet 2001;358:527-33). Based on these results, the ACC/AHA guidelines were updated to recommend that patients with ACS (unstable angina or non-ST-elevation MI) receive clopidogrel for 9 months in addition to aspirin and other standard therapies (J Am Coll Cardiol 2002;40:1366-74).

b. **Adjunct to elective PCI for patients with coronary artery disease.** In the Clopidogrel for the Reduction of Events During Observation (CREDO) trial, 2116 patients undergoing elective PCI were randomized to long-term (1-year) therapy with aspirin plus clopidogrel vs. short-term (4-week) therapy with aspirin plus clopidogrel followed by aspirin alone. At 1 year, long-term therapy resulted in a 26.9% relative reduction in the combined endpoint of death, MI, or stroke (p = 0.02) (JAMA 2002;288:2411-20). Also noted was a nonsignificant 25% relative risk reduction in stroke.

    c. **Prevention of recurrent stroke and other vascular events in patients with recent TIA or stroke.** The Management of ATherothrombosis with Clopidogrel in High-risk patients with recent TIA or ischemic stroke (MATCH) trial is comparing aspirin (75 mg/d) plus clopidogrel (75 mg/d) to clopidogrel alone (75 m/d) in approximately 7600 patients with recent (< 3 months) TIA or ischemic stroke and high risk of recurrent ischemic events (prior ischemic stroke, prior MI, angina pectoris, peripheral arterial disease, or diabetes). The combined endpoint is MI, stroke, vascular death, or rehospitalization for ischemic events during 18 months follow-up. The study has completed enrollment, and results will be available in early 2004. The CHARISMA trial will evaluate the combination of aspirin (75-162 mg/d) plus clopidogrel (75 mg/d) vs. aspirin alone (75-162 mg/d) in 15,200 patients at high atherothrombotic risk (primary and secondary prevention), including patients with previous TIA, ischemic stroke, or carotid stenosis. The primary endpoint of CHARISMA is first occurrence of either cardiovascular death, nonfatal MI, or nonfatal stroke. Results are expected in 2006.

C. Summary (Figure 10.3). All patients with prior ischemic TIA or stroke due to large artery atherothrombosis should receive antiplatelet therapy unless there is a specific contraindication. Monotherapy with aspirin (75-325 mg/d), clopidogrel (75 mg/d), or ticlopidine (250 mg bid) reduces the risk of MI, stroke, or cardiovascular death by approximately 25% compared to placebo. Aspirin is the least expensive agent, while the thienopyridines (clopidogrel/ticlopidine) are more potent antiplatelet agents than aspirin. (Clopidogrel is better tolerated with fewer adverse effects than ticlopidine.) Compared to aspirin alone, dual antiplatelet therapy with low-dose aspirin plus extended-release dipyridamole (25 mg/200 mg bid) was more effective at reducing recurrent stroke in ESPS-2, but it did not reduce the risk of MI or death compared to either agent alone. Based on the results of CAPRIE, CURE, and CREDO, it is reasonable to consider treating patients with prior ischemic TIA or stroke with combination aspirin plus clopidogrel, particularly those at increased risk of cardiac events; further recommendations await the results of the MATCH trial.

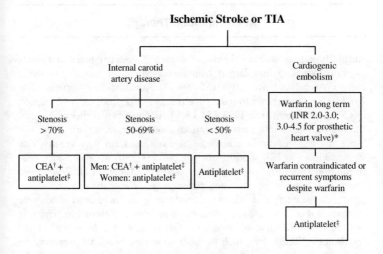

Figure 10.3. Antiplatelet and Antithrombotic Therapy for Secondary Prevention of Ischemic Stroke

INR = international normalized ratio, TIA = transient ischemic attack

* Consider aspirin 325 mg/d instead of warfarin for lone atrial fibrillation (age < 60 years and no hypertension, heart failure, mitral valve disease, prior embolism).

† Carotid endarterectomy can reduce the annual risk of stroke by 50% (from 2% per year to 1% per year) if performed by a surgeon with morbidity/mortality rate < 3%. Carotid stenting may be considered in select cases.

‡ Aspirin (325 mg/d), clopidogrel (75 mg/d), or combination low-dose aspirin plus extended-release dipyridamole (25mg/200mg bid). Consider combination aspirin (81-325 mg/d) plus clopidogrel (75 mg/d) for high-risk patients, especially those at increased risk of cardiac events. See discussion, pp. 77-85. For plaque disease some studies suggest benefit with lower-dose aspirin (81-165 mg/d).

Antithrombotic Therapy

Atrial fibrillation increases the risk of death by 2-fold compared to patients in normal sinus rhythm, largely from increased risk of stroke or systemic emboli (Arch Intern Med 1995;155:469-73). Adjusted-dose warfarin (INR 2.0-3.0) has been shown to reduce the risk of stroke from atrial fibrillation by 68% (Arch Intern Med. 1994;154:1449). All patients with rheumatic atrial fibrillation and without contraindications should receive warfarin long term. Since the risks of stroke and bleeding from warfarin vary greatly, risk stratification can help decide whether patients with nonrheumatic atrial fibrillation should receive aspirin or warfarin (Table 10.1). Warfarin is sometimes used in patients not undergoing revascularization of severe stenosis in the internal carotid or vertebral arteries and in patients with severe stenosis or recent occlusion of intracranial arteries. Antithrombin therapy is posited to be effective in conditions that promote the formation of red (erythrocyte-fibrin) clots, such as stasis within the heart, large protruding aortic atheromas, and severe stenosis or occlusion of large arteries. The routine addition of aspirin to low-dose warfarin has not been shown to confer any significant benefit over standard warfarin dosing with respect to stroke prevention. Recently, in SPORTIF-III, ximelagatran, an oral direct thrombin inhibitor, was shown to be at least as safe and effective as warfarin at preventing stroke in patients with nonvalvular AF, without the need for monitoring (p. 113); results of SPORTIF-V are pending.

Table 10.1. Stratification of Nonrheumatic Atrial Fibrillation

Biannual Stroke Risk	Patient Features	2001 ACCP Recommendations*	NNT to Prevent 1 Stroke
Low (approx. 2%)	Age < 65, no major risk factors[†]	Aspirin	227
Low moderate (approx. 3%)	Age 65-75, no major risk factors[†]	Aspirin or warfarin (INR 2-3)	Aspirin: 152 Warfarin: 54
High moderate (approx. 5%)	Age 65-75, no major risk factors[†] but with either diabetes or coronary disease	Warfarin (INR 2-3)	32
High (approx. 12%)	Age < 75 with hypertension, left ventricular dysfunction, or both, or age > 75 without other risk factors[†]	Warfarin (INR 2-3)	14
Very high (approx. 20%)	Age > 75 with hypertension, left ventricular dysfunction, or both, or any age and prior stroke, TIA, or systemic embolism	Warfarin (INR 2-3)	8

INR = international normalized ratio, NNT = number needed to treat, TIA = transient ischemic attack

*   Adapted from 2001 American College of Chest Physicians recommendations, which apply only to patients without contraindications to the suggested therapies

†   Major risk factors include: prior stroke, systemic embolism, or transient ischemic attack; hypertension; poor left ventricular function (clinical history or heart failure or ejection fraction < 50% on echocardiogram)

Adapted from: JAMA 2002;288:1388-1395

Chapter 11

Control of Hypertension

Hypertension affects 50 million Americans, including 60% of those over the age of 60. Each year, about 1.8 million new cases of hypertension develop, 75% of which are Stage 1 disease (140-159/90-99 mmHg). Among individuals aged 55-65 years without hypertension at baseline, the residual life-time risk of developing hypertension is 90% (JAMA 2002;287:1003-10). More than 90% of hypertension is idiopathic (essential), while 5-10% can be ascribed to an identifiable cause (secondary hypertension). Essential hypertension is caused by increased vascular reactivity and/or the inappropriate renal retention of salt and water. Over many years, this leads to accelerated atherosclerosis in large vessels, obliterative changes and/or thinning and rupture of small vessels, and increased workload on the heart.

Hypertension is the most important modifiable risk factor for stroke. Severe hypertension increases the risk of stroke by 7-fold, and borderline hypertension increases the risk by 1.5-fold. An average reduction of 9/5 mmHg can reduce the risk of stroke by 35-45% within 2-3 years of therapy (Lancet 2001;358:1033-41; Lancet 2000;355:865-72; Lancet 1991;338:1281; Lancet 1990;335:827), and benefits extend to patients > 80 years of age (Lancet 1999;353:793-796). Proper treatment reduces by 30% the incidence and fatality from coronary heart disease, heart failure, and kidney disease. Despite these beneficial effects, hypertension is grossly underdiagnosed and undertreated: only 68% of adults with hypertension are aware of their condition, only 50% are receiving medications, and only 27% of treated patients have blood pressures < 140/90 mmHg. Thiazide diuretics, beta-blockers, ACE inhibitors, and long-acting dihydropyridine calcium antagonists have all been shown to reduce the risk of stroke (CMAJ 1999;161:25-32; JAMA 1997;277:739-45; Lancet 2000;356:1955-65; Am J Med 2001;111:553-8).

Diagnosis and Evaluation of Hypertension

Hypertension is defined by a systolic blood pressure ≥ 140 mmHg ± diastolic blood pressure ≥ 90 mmHg, based on the average of two or more readings at two or more visits after the initial screen. A single recording may be sufficient if systolic blood pressure is ≥ 210 mmHg or diastolic blood pressure is ≥ 120 mmHg, especially if symptoms are present, but even very high elevations in blood pressure may occur transiently during extreme stress or acute illness. Blood pressure ≥ 135/85 mmHg outside the physician's office should also be considered elevated.

A. **Proper Blood Pressure Measurement Technique.** Improper technique can result in the overdiagnosis or underdiagnosis of hypertension (Table 11.1). Up to 50% of patients found to have elevated blood pressure on initial exam will not have persistently elevated blood pressures. Blood pressure measurements should be repeated over weeks to months to ensure that hypertension is present and persistent.

   1. **Have the patient sit quietly** for at least 5 minutes in a chair with back supported and arm supported at heart level, either passively or by a table. Standing, sitting unsupported, or actively holding the arm at heart level can raise blood pressure by 5-10 mmHg.

   2. **Ensure no caffeine or smoking** within the last 30-60 minutes and no recent use of exogenous adrenergic stimulants (e.g., phenylephrine in nasal decongestants); these can elevate blood pressure.

   3. **Use an appropriate size cuff.** The bladder should encircle about 80% of the arm circumference. If arm circumference is > 33 cm, a large cuff must be used to avoid artificially high readings.

   4. **Apply the cuff** so that the lower margin is 2-3 cm above the antecubital space. Ensure the middle of the bladder overlies the brachial artery pulse.

   5. **Inflate the bladder quickly** ~ 20 mmHg above systolic pressure (i.e., disappearance of radial pulse). Ensure the arm cuff is at the level of the heart.

   6. **Deflate the bladder at 2-3 mmHg per second**, recording pressures at both the beginning and disappearance of the Korotkoff sounds. More rapid deflation can underestimate systolic pressure and

overestimate diastolic pressure.

7. **Wait 1-2 minutes and repeat the measurement.** A third reading should be obtained if the variance exceeds 5 mmHg.

8. **Other tips**: If pressures differ between arms, the higher reading should be used. If arm pressure is elevated, a leg pressure should be measured, especially in younger patients, to detect coarctation of the aorta. For patients with atrial fibrillation or frequent extrasystoles, the average of several measurements should be recorded. It is important to check for orthostatic changes before and after initiating/increasing drug therapy, especially in diabetics and the elderly, and in patients with lightheadedness or dizziness. Ambulatory monitoring and frequent home measurements are often helpful in quantifying blood pressure abnormalities.

Table 11.1. Factors Affecting Blood Pressure Recordings

Overestimates True BP		Underestimates True BP	No Effect on BP
Examinee	**Examiner**	**Examinee**	**Examinee**
Soft Korotkoff sounds (diastolic BP effect)	Expectation bias	Soft Korotkoff sounds (systolic BP effect)	Menstrual phase
	Impaired hearing		Chronic caffeine
	Examination	Recent meal	Phenylephrine
Pseudohypertension	Cuff too narrow	Missed auscultatory gap	nasal spray
White-coat reaction	Cuff not centered	High stroke volume	Cuff self-inflation
Paretic arm (stroke)	Cuff over	**Setting, equipment**	**Examination**
Pain, anxiety	clothing	Noisy environment	Thin shirtsleeve
Acute smoking	Elbow too low	Faulty aneroid device	under cuff
Acute caffeine	Cuff too low	Low mercury level	Bell vs.
Acute ethanol	Short rest period	Leaky bulb	diaphragm
Distended bladder	Back	**Examiner**	Cuff inflation
Talking, signing	unsupported	Reading to next lowest 5	Hour of day
Setting, equipment	Arm unsupported	or 10 mmHg	Room
Environment noise	Too slow/fast	Expectation bias	temperature
Leaky bulb valve	deflation	Impaired hearing	
Blocked manometer		**Examination**	
Cold hands or		Left vs. right arm	
stethoscope		Resting too long	
		Elbow too high	
		Too rapid deflation	
		Excess bell pressure	

Adapted from: JAMA 1995;273:1211-1218

B. Excluding Conditions Leading to Overdiagnosis of Hypertension

    1. White-Coat Hypertension. White-coat hypertension is defined as hypertension that occurs only during doctors office visits and accounts for ≥ 20% of apparent hypertension (JAMA 1988;259:225-8). The diagnosis should be suspected in patients with persistent elevations in blood pressure but without evidence of target organ damage and is confirmed by ambulatory and home monitoring with measurements consistently ≤ 135/85 mmHg. Over 10 years, white-coat hypertension is associated with little if any increased risk of end-organ damage (Circulation 1998;98:1892-97). Treatment consists of lifestyle modifications and close follow-up. Drug therapy is reserved for patients with persistent hypertension.

    2. Pseudohypertension. Pseudohypertension occurs when the blood pressure cuff pressure needed to completely compress an extremely calcified and rigid brachial artery greatly exceeds intra-arterial pressure; this results in artificial elevations in blood pressure. Pseudohypertension should be suspected in elderly patients with generalized atherosclerosis; in patients whose radial artery can still be palpated when cuff pressure exceeds auscultatory systolic blood pressure (Osler's sign); and in patients with elevated blood pressure who develop hypotensive symptoms on drug therapy.

C. Assessment of Target Organ Damage. All hypertensive patients should be evaluated for target organ damage and clinical cardiovascular disease, including: cerebrovascular disease (TIAs, stroke); cardiovascular disease (angina, prior MI or coronary revascularization, heart failure, left ventricular hypertrophy); retinopathy (hemorrhages, exudates, papilledema); nephropathy (increased creatinine, proteinuria, microalbuminuria); peripheral artery disease (claudication, aneurysm, absent or diminished arterial pulses).

D. Detection of Secondary Hypertension. Hypertension ascribed to an identifiable cause represents 5% of the total hypertensive population. Indications for work-up include: (1) clinical features suggesting a secondary cause (Table 11.2); (2) resistance to triple drug therapy; (3) blood pressure worsening after a period of good control; (4) accelerated or malignant hypertension; or (5) negative family history with diastolic blood pressure > 110 mmHg.

Table 11.2. Causes of Secondary Hypertension

Cause	Features
Renovascular hypertension	Age < 30 years or > 60 years, diastolic pressure ≥ 120 mmHg, recent onset or exacerbation of hypertension (< 2 years), malignant hypertension, systolic-diastolic bruit in upper abdomen, refractory hypertension, acquired resistance to antihypertensive therapy (especially in elderly patients), deterioration in renal function after ACE inhibitors or angiotensin II receptor blockers
Pheochromo-cytoma	Spells of headache, palpitations, tachycardia, inappropriate perspiration, tremor, pallor; unusually labile blood pressure; recent weight loss; recent onset diabetes; malignant hypertension; pressor response to antihypertensive drugs or during induction of anesthesia; refractory hypertension. Symptoms are usually but not necessarily paroxysmal
Hyperthyroid-ism	Palpitations, tremor, weight loss, sweating, increased appetite
Primary aldosteronism	Unprovoked hypokalemia with inappropriate kaliuresis (24-hour urinary potassium ≥ 40 mEq with serum potassium ≤ 3.5 mEq/L), refractory hypertension
Cushing's syndrome	Truncal obesity, moon facies, ecchymosis, striae, acne, hirsutism, muscle weakness, osteoporosis, glucose intolerance, hypokalemia
Coarctation of the aorta	Absent, delayed, or diminished arterial pulsations in lower extremities, especially in patients < 30 years of age
Medications	Birth control pills, amphetamines (diet pills, cold capsules, nasal spray), MAO inhibitors, tricyclic antidepressants, cocaine, adrenal steroids, exogenous thyroid hormone, cyclosporine, erythropoietin
Others	Renal parenchymal disease, alcohol > 2 oz. per day, acromegaly, hypothyroidism, hypercalcemia (hyperparathyroidism), congenital adrenal hyperplasia, pregnancy-induced, neurological disorders (increased intracranial pressure, sleep apnea, quadriplegia, acute porphyria, familial dysautonomia, lead poisoning, Guillain-Barre syndrome), acute stress, systolic hypertension (aortic insufficiency, AV fistula, patent ductus arteriosus, thyrotoxicosis, Paget's disease, beriberi, rigidity of aorta)

Treatment of Hypertension

A. **Blood Pressure Goals.** The goal of blood pressure control is to reduce disability and death associated with hypertension using the least intrusive means. As shown in Table 11.3 and Figure 11.1, blood pressure should be reduced to < 140/90 mmHg for the general population and to < 130/80 mmHg in patients with diabetes or chronic renal disease. It is now known that *systolic* blood pressure, not diastolic blood pressure, is the major risk and goal of therapy. To achieve maximum benefit, systolic and diastolic blood pressures should be reduced to established targets.

Table 11.3. Initial Treatment of Hypertension

Blood Pressure Classification (systolic/diastolic BP, mmHg)*	Lifestyle Modification	Initial Drug Therapy**
Normal (< 120 and < 80)	-	-
Prehypertension (120-139 or 80-89)	Yes	For compelling indication[†]
Stage 1 (140-159 or 90-99)	Yes	1- or 2-drug therapy
Stage 2 (≥ 160/100)	Yes	2-drug therapy for most

*   When systolic and diastolic pressures fall into different categories, the higher category should be used to classify blood pressure status (e.g., 160/92 mmHg should be classified as stage 2 hypertension). Isolated systolic hypertension is defined by a systolic BP of ≥ 140 mmHg with a diastolic BP < 90 mmHg and should be staged appropriately (e.g., 170/85 mmHg is defined as stage 2 isolated systolic hypertension)

**   BP goal < 140/90 mmHg. For patients with diabetes or chronic kidney disease, treat to BP < 130/80 mmHg. Treat with thiazide diuretic, ACE inhibitor, angiotensin receptor blocker, beta-blocker, calcium antagonist, or combination drug therapy, depending on patient characteristics (e.g., African-Americans, elderly), coexistent medical conditions (e.g., diabetes, chronic renal disease), and level of blood pressure. Start 2 drugs in most patients with BP > 20/10 mmHg above target BP

†   For patients with diabetes mellitus or chronic kidney disease, treat to BP < 130/80 mmHg

Adapted from: The Seventh Report of the Joint National Committee on Prevention, Detection, Evaluation, and Treatment of High Blood Pressure (JAMA 2003;289:2560-72).

High Blood Pressure

Begin or Continue Lifestyle Modifications

- Lose weight if overweight
- Limit alcohol to no more than 2 drinks/day (1 oz or 30 mL of ethanol [24 oz beer, 10 oz wine, or 3 oz 80-proof whiskey) in most men and no more than 1 drink/day in women and lighter-weight persons
- Increase aerobic physical activity to 30-45 minutes most days of the week
- Reduce sodium intake to ≤ 100 mmol/d (2.4 gm/d sodium or 6 gm/d sodium chloride)
- Maintain adequate intake of dietary potassium (~ 90 mmol/d), calcium, magnesium
- Stop smoking for overall cardiovascular health
- Increase dietary intake of fruits, vegetables, and low-fat dairy with a reduced content of saturated fat and total fat

---

Not at Blood Pressure Goal
General population: < 140/90 mmHg
Diabetes mellitus or chronic kidney disease: < 130/80 mmHg

Initiate Drug Therapy*
Initiate drug therapy based on patient characteristics, coexistent conditions, and BP level
Start 2 drugs in most patients with BP > 20/10 mmHg above target BP

Not at Blood Pressure Goal

Optimize dosages or add additional drugs until BP goal is achieved
Consider referral to a hypertension specialist

Figure 11.2. Treatment of Hypertension

*   Drug therapy is often initiated concurrently with lifestyle modification in high-risk patients

Adapted from: The Seventh Report of the Joint National Committee on Prevention, Detection, Evaluation, and Treatment of High Blood Pressure (JAMA 2003;289:2560-72).

B. Drug Therapy

1. **Initial Therapy.** The choice of initial drug therapy should be individualized, based on patient characteristics, associated medical conditions, and blood pressure levels. In general, most patients should be started on a low dose of a long-acting once-daily drug that can be titrated slowly based on the patient's age and response (e.g, every 1-2 months for Stage 1 hypertension). About 50% of patients respond to monotherapy. In high-risk patients (BP ≥ 180/110 mmHg, clinical cardiovascular disease, target organ damage), intervals between adding new drugs and changing existing regimens can be reduced. If BP is > 20/10 mmHg above target BP, it is reasonable to initiate therapy with 2 drugs, one of which should usually be a thiazide-type diuretic (JAMA 2003;289:2560-72). Hospitalization should be considered for persons with blood pressures ≥ 200/120 mmHg and symptomatic target organ damage.

2. **Intensification of Therapy.** The sequence for intensification of drug therapy depends on the response to and tolerance of initial therapy. If the initial drug has no effect on blood pressure or causes bothersome side effects, another drug from a different drug class should be substituted. If a partial response is obtained and the drug is well tolerated, a higher dose can be given or a second agent from a different drug class can be added. (If a diuretic is not chosen as initial therapy, it should probably be added next, as it will enhance the effect of most antihypertensive drugs.) If target blood pressure is still not attained, continue adding drugs from other classes. Before proceeding to each successive treatment step, examine potential reasons for lack of responsiveness, including pseudohypertension (p. 91), nonadherence to therapy, volume overload, drug-related causes, and secondary causes of hypertension. Elevated blood pressure alone in asymptomatic patients without new or worsening target organ damage rarely requires emergency control.

3. **Combination Drug Therapy.** Once-daily, fixed-dose combination therapy, in which a full dose of one drug is replaced by smaller doses of two or more drugs, is a common approach for initial treatment of hypertension. The different mechanisms of action may result in fewer side effects and better blood pressure control, especially in the

resistant hypertensive. For the 60% of patients and 75% of diabetics who require more than one antihypertensive drug, once-daily, fixed-dose combination therapy may improve compliance. Useful combinations include a diuretic plus either a beta-blocker, calcium antagonist, ACE inhibitor, or angiotensin II receptor blocker; an ACE inhibitor plus a calcium antagonist; an ACE inhibitor plus eplerenone (aldosterone receptor blocker); a diuretic plus an adrenergic blocker plus a vasodilator; or a beta-blocker plus a calcium antagonist. Combinations that should be avoided include two drugs from the same class (e.g., two beta-blockers); a centrally-acting agent and a beta-blocker; and a beta-blocker plus either diltiazem or verapamil. In the PROGRESS trial, combination therapy with perindopril plus indapamide reduced blood pressure by 12/5 mmHg and recurrent stroke by 43% (p. 129).

4. **Stepdown Therapy.** Monotherapy ultimately provides adequate blood pressure control for ~ 50% of patients. Therefore, if blood pressure has been well-controlled on two drugs for ≥ 6 months, gradual withdrawal of the first drug may be attempted. Close monitoring is advised since hypertension may return after a delayed period of months to years. Attempts to completely discontinue antihypertensive therapy are generally not recommended without sustained and substantial improvements in lifestyle.

D. **Optimizing Patient Compliance.** Since 50% or more of hypertensive patients adjust or discontinue antihypertensive therapy on their own, education about dietary, lifestyle, and pharmacologic measures is essential. Drugs should be chosen that are affordable, treat coexistent disease, and have convenient dosing and favorable side-effect profiles. Patients should also be educated about the silent nature of the disease and its risks if left untreated. Adherence to antihypertensive therapy can also be improved by challenging patients to play an active role in their disease—recording blood pressure at home, reporting side effects, involving their families, challenging them to reach and maintain the therapeutic goal. Patients should also be encouraged to record and report their blood pressure prior to their morning drug dose (to ensure protection against the surge in blood pressure upon awakening) and in the early evening (to ensure coverage throughout the day). Compliance measures should be reinforced at every visit.

Chapter 12

Control of Dyslipidemia

Elevated plasma levels of total cholesterol and LDL cholesterol and low plasma levels of HDL cholesterol are major modifiable lipid risk factors for atherothrombotic vascular disease. It has been estimated that for each 1% decrease in LDL cholesterol and for each 1% increase in HDL cholesterol, the risk for cardiovascular events falls by 2% and 3%, respectively. A meta-analysis of more than 30 trials using diet, drugs (including statins), or surgery to lower cholesterol has shown that for every 1% total cholesterol is lowered, total mortality is reduced by 1.1% (Circulation 1995;91:2274-82; Circulation 1998;97:946-52). Large randomized trials (CARE, LIPID, 4S) have shown that statins reduce the risk of stroke by 25-35% in patients with hyperlipidemia as well as those with previous MI and relatively normal cholesterol levels. In the Heart Protection Study, the largest statin study to date, 20,536 patients with atherosclerotic arterial disease or diabetes were randomized to simvastatin 40 mg or placebo. At 5 years, statin therapy reduced the risk of first occurrence of non-fatal or fatal stroke by 25% (4.3% vs. 5.7%, $p < 0.0001$). Cardiac mortality, MI, and revascularization procedures were reduced by 18%, 38%, and 22%, respectively. The level of risk reduction with statins is similar to that achieved with aspirin for patients at high risk of stroke. The beneficial effects of lipid therapy are due more to plaque stabilization than to changes in stenosis severity, which are generally modest and disproportionate to the 25-80% reduction in major vascular events. Plaque stabilization, which can be accomplished in weeks to months with aggressive treatment of dyslipidemia, may be related to resorption of macrophage and extracellular lipid deposits, a decrease in neointimal inflammation, and maintenance of fibrous cap integrity. Effective treatment transforms the inflamed, friable plaque into a stable, fibrotic plaque that is less prone to ulceration, rupture, and thrombosis. In addition, lipid-lowering therapy improves endothelial dysfunction caused by dyslipidemia, resulting in additional vasodilatory, antithrombotic, and anti-inflammatory effects.

Diagnosis, Evaluation, and Treatment of Dyslipidemia

A. **Lipoprotein Analysis.** A fasting lipoprotein profile consisting of total cholesterol, LDL cholesterol, HDL cholesterol, and triglyceride should be obtained in all adults over age 20 and repeated at least once every 5 years. If a nonfasting test is performed, only total cholesterol and HDL cholesterol measurements are reliable. Blood samples should be drawn after a 9-12 hour fast while the person is in a steady state (absence of active weight loss, acute illness, recent trauma or surgery, pregnancy, or recent change in diet).

B. **Exclusion of Secondary Causes.** Once a dyslipidemia is identified, a history, physical examination, and basic laboratory tests are performed to screen for secondary causes of dyslipidemia, including diet, medications, alcohol abuse, diabetes, hypothyroidism, nephrotic syndrome, chronic renal failure, and obstructive liver disease.

C. **Identification of Genetic Dyslipidemia.** If severe hypercholesterolemia is present (total cholesterol > 300 mg/dL) or a genetic disorder is discovered, a family history and measurement of cholesterol in other family members are needed.

D. **LDL and Non-HDL Cholesterol Goals.** LDL lowering is the primary goal of therapy for persons with dyslipidemia, and LDL goals vary inversely with CHD risk: individuals at highest risk have the lowest LDL targets. Non-HDL cholesterol (i.e., LDL + VLDL cholesterol, calculated by subtracting HDL cholesterol from total cholesterol) is a secondary goal of therapy after LDL lowering in persons with triglycerides ≥ 200 mg/dL. LDL and non-HDL goals are shown in Table 12.1.

E. **Metabolic Syndrome.** Many persons have a constellation of major and emerging risk factors, referred to as the metabolic syndrome, that increase the risk of coronary and cerebrovascular events at any level of LDL cholesterol. These individuals benefit from specific therapeutic measures beyond LDL lowering. Clinical identification of the metabolic syndrome requires ≥ 3 of the following factors: abdominal obesity (waist circumference: men > 102 cm [40 in]; women > 88 cm [35 in]);

triglycerides ≥ 150 mg/dL; low HDL cholesterol (men < 40 mg/dL; women < 50 mg/dL); blood pressure ≥ 130/85 mmHg; impaired fasting glucose (fasting glucose 110-125 mg/dL)

Table 12.1. LDL and Non-HDL Cholesterol Goals

Risk Category	LDL Goal (mg/dL)	Non-HDL Goal* (mg/dL)
CHD or CHD risk equivalent (10-yr risk for CHD > 20%[‡])	< 100	< 130
≥ 2 risk factors[†] with 10-yr risk for CHD ≤ 20%[‡]	< 130	< 160
0-1 risk factor[†]	< 160	< 190

CHD = coronary heart disease, CHD risk equivalent = carotid artery disease (TIA or stroke of carotid origin, asymptomatic carotid stenosis > 50%); peripheral vascular disease (including abdominal aortic aneurysm); other atherosclerotic vascular disease (e.g., renal artery stenosis); diabetes mellitus; or ≥ 2 risk factors conferring 10-year CHD risk > 20%

*   To determine non-HDL cholesterol, subtract HDL cholesterol from total cholesterol. Non-HDL cholesterol is a secondary goal of therapy after LDL lowering for persons with triglycerides ≥ 200 mg/dL

[†]   Major risk factors that modify LDL goal include: cigarette smoking; hypertension (BP ≥ 140/90 mmHg or on antihypertensive medication); low HDL cholesterol (< 40 mg/dL); family history of premature CHD (CHD in male first-degree relative < 55 years; CHD in female first-degree relative < 65 years); age (men ≥ 45 years; women ≥ 55 years)

[‡]   As determined by the Framingham risk score (Circulation 2002;106:3145-3421)

Treatment of Elevated LDL Cholesterol

Therapeutic lifestyle changes (diet, physical activity, weight control, smoking cessation) are considered first-line therapy for all patients with dyslipidemia. Drug therapy should be initiated on the initial visit concurrently with lifestyle changes in high-risk persons, including those with prior TIA or stroke or asymptomatic carotid stenosis > 50% (Figure 12.1).

Elevated LDL Cholesterol

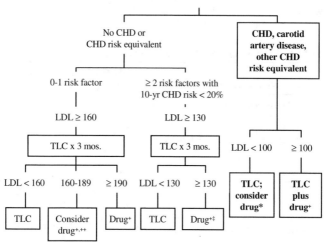

Figure 12.1. Treatment of Elevated LDL Cholesterol

LDL levels are expressed in mg/dL. CHD = coronary heart disease; CHD risk equivalent = carotid artery disease (TIA or stroke of carotid origin; asymptomatic carotid stenosis > 50%), abdominal aortic aneurysm, peripheral arterial disease, diabetes mellitus, or multiple (≥ 2) risk factors with 10-year CHD risk > 20%; CHD risk factors = see footnotes, Table 12.1. TLC = therapeutic lifestyle changes (Chapters 8-13)

*   Consider statin therapy, based on results of the Heart Protection Study (p. 134)

+   Initial drug therapy usually consists of moderate dose of a statin. If LDL cholesterol at 6 weeks remains above the LDL target, options include: (1) intensify diet therapy by adding plant sterols/stanols 2 gm/day and increasing soluble fiber to 10-25 gm/d); (2) intensify statin therapy; (3) consider adding a bile acid sequestrant, niacin, or ezetimibe; (4) if elevated triglyceride or low HDL is present, consider adding nicotinic acid or a fibrates to statin therapy; or (5) if LDL is near target, consider maintaining current statin dose. Difficult-to-control patients should be referred to a lipid specialist

++ Especially consider drug therapy for individuals with at least 1 strong risk factor (severe hypertension, heavy cigarette smoker, family history of premature CHD)

‡   Drug therapy is recommended for persons with a 10-year risk of CHD of 10-20%. If 10-year risk is < 10%, drug therapy is optional but may be especially useful in individuals with at least 1 strong risk factor (severe hypertension, heavy cigarette smoker, strong family history of premature CHD)

Treatment of Low HDL Cholesterol
and Elevated Triglyceride

A. Low HDL Cholesterol. HDL is involved in reverse cholesterol transport from the peripheral tissues to the liver. A depressed HDL cholesterol level (< 40 mg/dL) is a powerful predictor of vascular risk. Causes of low HDL cholesterol include elevated triglycerides, obesity, physical inactivity, cigarette smoking, very high carbohydrate diets (> 60% of calories), type 2 diabetes, drugs (beta-blockers, anabolic steroids, progestational agents), and genetic factors. Nonpharmacologic measures that increase HDL cholesterol include weight loss, exercise, and smoking cessation. Diets high in monounsaturated and omega-3 fatty acids can also increase HDL cholesterol without increasing LDL cholesterol. Alcohol increases HDL cholesterol but is not recommended for that purpose. Once LDL and non-HDL goals are achieved, drug therapy to raise HDL cholesterol may be considered for higher-risk individuals (Figure 12.2).

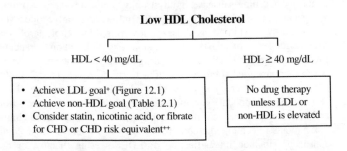

Low HDL Cholesterol

HDL < 40 mg/dL

- Achieve LDL goal+ (Figure 12.1)
- Achieve non-HDL goal (Table 12.1)
- Consider statin, nicotinic acid, or fibrate for CHD or CHD risk equivalent++

HDL ≥ 40 mg/dL

No drug therapy unless LDL or non-HDL is elevated

Figure 12.2. Treatment of Low HDL Cholesterol

See Figure 12.1 for abbreviations
+   Statin is preferred drug therapy
++ For individuals without CHD and 1 or more risk factors, drug therapy can be considered for higher-risk persons with asymptomatic atherosclerosis by coronary EBCT or arterial neck ultrasound

B. Elevated Triglyceride. Elevated triglyceride is an independent risk factor for coronary disease and is associated with atherogenic VLDL remnants and small dense LDL particles, which correlate with the extent and progression of atherosclerosis. ATP III defines normal triglyceride as < 150 mg/dL, borderline-high triglyceride as 200-499 mg/dL, and very high triglyceride as ≥ 500 mg/dL. Since remnant lipoproteins are comprised of partially degraded VLDL particles, elevated VLDL cholesterol levels can be used as a marker for the presence of remnant lipoproteins and elevated risk. ATP III recognizes non-HDL cholesterol (LDL + VLDL cholesterol) as a secondary target of therapy in patients with high triglyceride (≥ 200 mg/dL) and sets the non-HDL goal at 30 mg/dL higher than the LDL goal (Table 12.1), based on the assumption that higher VLDL levels are associated with remnant lipoproteins and increased vascular risk. Non-HDL cholesterol is determined by subtracting HDL cholesterol from total cholesterol. Causes of elevated triglyceride include lifestyle-related causes (obesity, physical inactivity, cigarette smoking, excess alcohol intake, high carbohydrate diet), other secondary causes (diabetes mellitus, chronic renal failure, nephrotic syndrome, Cushing's disease, lipodystrophy, pregnancy, various drugs), and genetic causes. The potential benefits of lowering triglyceride levels are not as well studied as those of lowering LDL cholesterol. For triglyceride levels of 150-199 mg/dL, emphasis is placed on therapeutic lifestyle changes and LDL lowering; drug therapy to reduce triglycerides is not recommended (Figure 12.3). For triglyceride levels of 200-499 mg/dL, primary therapy is directed at LDL lowering, and non-HDL cholesterol is a secondary goal of therapy. In addition to weight reduction and increased physical activity, drug therapy may be considered in high-risk patients to achieve the non-HDL cholesterol goal. Pharmacologic approaches include intensification of LDL-lowering therapy, or the addition of nicotinic acid or fibrates when used with appropriate caution. For very high triglyceride levels (≥ 500 mg/dL), the primary goal of therapy is to prevent acute pancreatitis by rapidly lowering triglycerides to < 500 mg/dL with very low fat diets (≤ 15% of calories), weight reduction, increased physical activity, and the use of either a fibrate or nicotinic acid. Once triglycerides are < 500 mg/dL, attention is directed toward achieving LDL cholesterol and non-HDL cholesterol targets.